Contents

To everyone who fears their dreams will be taken away for who they are, this is for you.

This book and the research that informs it are the conclusion of a long journey and internal dialogue. I grew up immersed in sports; it was a way for me to make new friends and to stay active. More than anything, it was a way to keep me away from video games and other screens that would come to dominate my time once I started using computers for research and other academic purposes. Growing up I understood that in some ways, I was very different from my peers. As my teammates and I grew up and become more aware of ourselves, they became more interested in the opposite gender and I found that I just did not have that kind of interest in girls that they did. Age and the internet finally gave me a queer identity, and while it was important for me to have that identity and to cherish it, that separation from the rest of society served to make me feel lonely. I began to wonder whether there was anyone else like me who played sports that I could bond with and share the experience of athletics with, particularly once I got near the end of my high school career and the terms used to attack opponents became increasingly derogatory and based on perceived sexuality. It was difficult for me to reconcile my own experiences in athletics, which I believe were truly and nearly entirely positive experiences with the fact that there was no one else in the leagues I played in that seemed to identify the same way. Even after I started coming out to my teammates, there was still no one who understood the things I was going through and that bothered me on a personal level and on a sociocultural level.

This genesis of a question of where queer athletes existed in youth athletics was one that I gave consideration to as a younger student, but not something that became a topic of research until very recently. Social media provided my initial impetus for researching queer issues in youth athletics; I had seen that one of my former teammates had come out of the closet and had been surprised that they did not come out to me while we had been teammates. I had been sure to come out to them while we played, and I could not understand why they would not invite me into their confidence when it was a secret we both shared. It was then that I decided that this was a phenomenon that needed to be studied in greater detail, this need to remain secretive in athletics as a queer person, and why there might be a perception that existed in athletics that would indicate queer people would not have been accepted if we were open about who we were. This perception that seemed to be in existence was in contrast to my own experiences in coming out and participating at various levels of athletics, which led to the main theme of the research. Just how homophobic and transphobic did youth think athletics were, and how much did those perceptions track with the actual experiences of participants.

The research done to complete this book was meant to determine how athletic organizations could reach youth who are otherwise concerned about facing a discriminatory or adversarial environment and engaging them in athletics. Queer issues are specifically highlighted in the research, with potential solutions and ideas for changing the way sports are marketed towards queer youth being tested through the research to determine how effective those ideas may be in enticing more youth to take part in sports, and what other problems would be faced by queer youth wanting to participate in athletics that might not otherwise be faced by cisgendered, heterosexual youth. My own personal experiences informed the remainder of the work that went into creating this book, and is based on addressing what I believe are critical flaws in the way Canadian society trains its coaches and prepares them for working with diverse populations of youth, some of whom will have challenges that fall outside the life experience of the coach and need to be part of the training programmes that coaches go through in order to best work with their charges.

I would like to express my very great appreciation to Doctor Joy Butler, without whom this project would never have begun. The advice you gave me at all steps of the process were instrumental in the completion of the research that spawned this book, and it was your help that ensured the project would succeed.

Advice given by Ms. Misha Dhillon for her initial encouragements to pursue this project, and also for her support and troubleshooting during the initial phases of the project. Your friendship and advice was especially important to me while obtaining ethics approval for this project.

Finally, a word of thanks to my parents, who encouraged me to complete this project and to do this work for the sake of doing this work, not knowing where it would lead me. I would never have done this if you had not believed in the need for this research and your belief in me to thoroughly research this topic.

Years of participating in competitive athletics left me with a conundrum; how to reconcile my identity as a gay male with my external identity as a competitive athlete? The concept of openly queer athletes was not even considered when I was actively engaged in competitive athletics, and indeed it was still at a point in history where being openly queer at all was still seen as different and even deviant.

Canadian society had not yet begun giving queer individuals legal rights and protections when I began to understand my sexual identity was going to be different from the vast majority of my peers. At the same time I was coming to terms with the fact that I was different, I was also becoming aware of the stereotypes that were commonly attributed to queer individuals. Without realising it at the time I had begun to question those stereotypes because of how poorly they reflected my own life, and soon after I began to wonder who among my teammates and opponents shared the same secret I had.

Since then I've come out to most of the teams I've played for, over a multitude of different sports. The question still hadn't been answered through research done by other scholars in the field and it was becoming clear that there had to be more than myself representing queer people in organized athletics.

I firmly believe that athletics is something that all people should have an opportunity to participate in and that doing so promotes healthier lifestyles and greater social connectedness with an individual's community. To that end, I wanted to determine what it was that was holding queer youth back from participating in athletics, and I devised a research proposal to probe some of the questions that were potential causes of lower rates of participation in athletics by queer youth.

With increasing numbers of professional and collegiate athletes coming out in highly publicized ways that are reaching youth across North America, I wanted to provide first-hand knowledge of how to come out to a sports team and provide advice to youth who were considering taking a similar path. There remains a significant set of hurdles that queer youth face before they can actively participate in athletics, and it is my hope that I will have addressed many of those concerns and provided potential solutions that can be used in regions and municipalities throughout the continent to ensure that everyone has the opportunity to play the sport they enjoy.

This book will provide insights into the policy creation process that can be used by athletes and their supporters to help create more responsive and queer-friendly policies in their own sports organizations and will serve to create stronger grassroots coalitions to protect the rights of all athletes to play without facing discrimination.

How does one compare the feeling of draining a last second three-pointer for a win? Catching the game winning touchdown in double-coverage? Sinking a forty-foot putt on the eighteenth for a win? Smashing a ball over the right field wall in extra innings? Asking an athlete to describe this feeling often evokes strong, emotionally loaded language; if the athlete is able to muster up words at all. Because in that moment...we are infinite. We are invincible. We are us. I believe in the poetic side of athletics. The raw beauty embedded in its core. Its ability to change people. Its ability to bring people together. Regardless of ideology...a field, court, course, whatever it is, it does not care about anything going on outside the moment. It is a comforting idea that for a set amount of time, nothing matters but the activity presented before you.

If you have experienced one of these speechless moments, you know how powerful and emotional of a feeling it is. Now imagine having all that stripped from you because of the gender you were attracted to. Something so trivial as sexual orientation defining your ability or inability to play a sport. It is nothing short of heartbreaking to imagine someone being deprived of something so beautiful and empowering as athletics because someone is not comfortable with who they are.

My name is Conner Mertens and I am the first active college football player to come out as LGBT at any level. In this process, I made my contact information available for anyone who could find it useful. All too often, the stories listed above were not a clever anecdote used to start a piece of writing, but the cruel reality for many athletes. The breakdown of people reaching out to me following my coming out was about twenty percent active athletes looking for support, twenty percent people of faith wanting to discuss that aspect and sixty percent former athletes with tales of discrimination and heartbreak. Email after email poured in with the words, "...and I forced to quit _____ because my team found out my sexual orientation." So imagine, if you will, all those incredible explanations of sport from earlier being ripped away from you. Not for lack of talent or ability but because someone else does not understand you. Criminal and gutwrenching is what that amounts to.

The fact that I was able to be open about my sexuality and not hide or suppress it was inconceivable by many of these former athletes. Fortunately for me, I found some amazing outlets and resources early on that helped make the process as smooth as it could be. Getting connected to the You Can Play Project immediately gave me confidence and comfort that I would not have had otherwise. However, without my initiative to actively go out and search for support, I would not have had that outlet. There seems to be a general lack of support for the LGBTQ athlete throughout sports. Without support for the LGBTQ athlete, we will continue hearing the very real stories of individuals forced to quit their respected sport for an issue that has absolutely nothing to do with athletics. We have comes leaps and bounds from Paragraph 175 in Nazi Germany and the Stonewall Riots in New York. But we still have a long ways to go.

In March of 2015, I spoke to a golfer at the Division 1 level who was kicked off their team the day after they were outed by teammates. This is shadowy reminder that these problems are not outdated nor abstract. This is a very real and very present issue that still requires our attention. I have seen the faces and heard the stories. The forceful end to one's athletic career because of their "lifestyle". Before I go on: let's quit referring to the existence of a demographic of people as a "lifestyle". It is me. Going to the gym is a lifestyle. Having love for someone is called being human. Another one is we need to stop praising individuals for their "tolerance". Tolerance is a small step up from hatred yet below indifference. Tolerance acknowledges that something or someone is not agreeable but that person is choosing to see past that inherent pitfall and put up with their existence. No one wants to be tolerated. People want to be loved and accepted. I tolerate broccoli, I love people.

At the end of the day, I am just a stupid kid. Thrown into the spotlight overnight for writing a letter to my hometown, I don't know much. But one thing I know and understand is the power and liberation behind the ability to simply be yourself. Friends from across all walks of life and demographics, take heed and hear these words (I've always wanted to say that)...they may even change your life. If you take nothing from my words, understand this: Bust out of that cage of oppression called insecurity and realize you were put on this earth not just to survive, but to thrive and be the best version of yourself. And above all else, know that hope is everywhere. You just have to know the right places to look.

I will leave you with this one simple question: Are you happy? Are you happy with what you are doing in this life? Are you living your life for yourself or for someone else? Have you lost track of who you are because it was easier being someone else? It took me many years to realize my own answer to these questions. I came out to one to one of my closest friends and they told me that I had given them the courage to finally tell that girl that he liked her. That's what this is about. Being real with yourself and others. If you like to dance, get jiggy wit it. If you like to sing, get your Justin Timberlake on. If you like to box, go get 'em, Rocky, if you like that girl, what's holding you back, Romeo. Point is, don't let society dictate who you can and cannot be simply because it doesn't fit their perception of who you are supposed to be.

I was finally starting to become free. Telling my teammates that I was gay and that I was still intending to remain a member of the team was a liberating experience and it made me a better player. The team, rather than shunning me or otherwise making me feel ostracized as an outsider who was different from the rest of them, reminded me that we were still all the same people and that what matters is what I do on the field, not off the field.

The first time I came out to a teammate of mine was just after my first year of midget level baseball. At that point I had been playing competitively for over a decade, and I had been playing with this particular team for three years. The problem was that I didn't feel like I was part of the team, and in a real sense I was not. My teammates were happy to talk about their relationships and I couldn't safely join the conversation without revealing my sexuality. This was something that I considered to be a risk to my safety, but at the same time I realized that I could not continue to hide the truth. It wasn't fair to my teammates and it made it more difficult for us all to connect.

Like most of my peers and many of the participants in this survey, I was convinced that there would be a negative backlash to my decision to come out and admit my sexuality to my teammates. Also like many of the participants in the research study, I was pleased to find that my fears had been unfounded and that my teammates did in fact grow closer to me once they had a better understanding of who I was and why I was so reluctant to open up at times. This did lead me to come out to other people and gave me more self-confidence in other areas of my life.

That was my coming out experience in the athletic world. Everyday, the athletes across the world are coming out and telling their teammates that they too are part of the queer continuum. Some will have experiences very similar to my own, while some will have far worse outcomes. Some queer youth will never have this experience at all, their fear of rejection and discrimination is too high to let them even consider athletics as a potential activity.

For most people, the idea of openly gay athletes is still a foreign one, a novelty that happens in other cities and towns, and never with their own children or their own teammates. There is a prevailing view that in exists in academia and the rest of the outside world that sports remains the last bastion of heteronormativity and homophobia, that sports are the realm of masculinity and conformity[i]. This was true in earlier decades, but those barriers are falling at an alarming rate thanks to work done at the professional level and grassroots organizations.

Youth in particular are beginning to understand that these attitudes are outdated, and have begun working in their communities and sports to change the face of athletics to become friendlier to queer athletes. Examples of these programs exist in almost every community in Canada and America, and yet there continues to be an unshakable belief among members of the queer community that sports are not welcoming to them[ii]. This research attempts to explain the reasoning behind those views, and what potential solutions there are to make athletics a welcoming place for all potential athletes.

The change in these attitudes is occurring at different rates throughout the world. The example of the recent Sochi Olympics has shown that there are still many nations and people who believe that queer people should have fewer rights and that the right place for queer people is at the margins of society[iii]. The signing of laws in Africa criminalizing homosexuality also serves to try and stigmatize queer individuals instead of providing safety for these members of the national community[iv].

On the other hand, the recent coming out of Michael Sam and the signing of Jason Collins to a professional contract in America speaks to the growing sense of acceptance that queer individuals are having in North America, and this in turn is having an impact on the younger generation[v]. Public opinion surveys consistently show that younger generations are more likely to be supportive of queer rights and further integration of queers into the national culture, which is now starting to penetrate into the national athletic psychology[vi].

The quantitative research done in this study is focused on the questions of the perceptions of youth, both queer-identifying and heterosexual, about the state of homophobia and transphobia in sports. In particular, the research attempts to identify the view of youth about different levels of sport and the acceptability of homophobia and transphobia at those levels of athletics. These questions about the youths' perceptions of athletics is compared with their lived experiences and present a conundrum for those who wish to increase youth athletic participation rates; how do sports enthusiasts get more queer youth involved when they are more likely to believe they will be discriminated against than their own experiences prove?

It is perhaps this point that is the most interesting; less than half the respondents, regardless of their gender identity or sexual orientation actually experienced or witnessed discrimination while participating, even as nearly two-thirds of the sample population were concerned about discrimination in sports and higher rates of respondents believed there were high levels of discrimination in sports.

Involvement in athletics has been shown to have medical and personal benefits, but it is important to note that participation rates and the ability to become involved is not even across Canada. Ethnicity, social class and gender continue to present barriers to participation, and naturally sexual orientation and gender identity are also strong barriers to participation in organized athletics. This continues to reflect the wider society, where male Caucasian heterosexuals of average income continue to hold a number of nontangible advantages over the rest of society. This continues in spite of policy changes and government action meant to ensure that minority groups have an equal or greater opportunity to achieve the same level of status and upward socio-economic mobility that is currently afforded to Caucasians.

In relating this to athletics, a cursory observation of professional sports shows that the vast majority of athletes are college graduates where they were drafted by their professional teams. Given that college attendance has historically been reserved for those with access to the funding to enrol, particularly in America, this is an indication that a certain socio-economic class dominates the athletic world at its highest levels. This is compounded by the fact that professional athletes in nearly every sport receive salaries that remain far above the national average in both Canada and the United States, such that whichever class an athlete may have started their life, once they become professionals they are very clearly a part of the upper class of society in terms of their personal wealth.

As is to be expected, the vast majority of individuals who participate in sports, even at the collegiate level, are unlikely to be selected to become professionals in their field. This process ensures that only those with the most natural talent and time available for intensive training are likely to be selected and serves as another means of reducing the likelihood of marginalized groups from participating and being included in professional athletics. While this is not true of all sports; witness the participation rates of African Americans in professional basketball and South Americans in professional baseball, it remains notable that nearly all sports leagues have a majority of their members composed of white males.

This brings us to our discussion of youth sports, and how certain groups continue to be over represented in athletics at the cost of other groups being able to participate. In most cases, this is not caused due to overt discrimination or policies putting quotas on the number of players from certain demographic groups. For youth athletics, the main consideration and barrier to participation remain the steep registration and insurance fees that leagues charge to allow youth to participate in sports. In the case of many sports, the fees are several hundred dollars in costs, and do not include other additional fees such as the costs of equipment and fuel to travel to games and practices. For more experienced teams or youth who participate in more rural environments, additional costs may also be incurred to cover the costs of overnight accommodations when travelling to games. These increased costs serve to make socio-economic class one of the major barriers to participating in athletics, ensuring that the majority of youth participants are middle class, and in Canada this has meant mostly that they are from either Caucasian or East

Asian backgrounds, with fewer participants from other ethnic backgrounds gaining participation into organized athletics.

Queer sexuality is one of the other main barriers to consideration of athletics, which this paper will address in greater detail. Those who identify as part of the queer community reported in this research greater concern about their safety, which are matched by their overall considerations of athletics as excessively homophobic and discriminatory. However, it should also be noted that the lack of participation in itself could be a cause for increased discrimination towards queer youth, particularly among males. It remains a social ideal that those who identify as male or are identified as male by society should be interested in participating in at least one athletic activity; the failure or lack of interest in doing so can often be seen as a strong reason to question the sexual orientation of the male that refuses to become involved in sports, and can sometimes perpetrate the very discrimination the youth was attempting to avoid by evading organized athletics.

What this has meant is that those who wish to succeed in sports have generally been winnowed away from participation for a variety of reasons, most of which are used to perpetrate the status quo of white male hegemony in society in general and athletics specifically. This has generally been seen as acceptable or at least tolerable for most athletes, professional organizations and athletic fans, who are more willing to pay ticket prices in order to view someone they can relate to on a demographic level.

The research conducted was a quantitative survey conducted over the course of eight months spanning from April 2013 to January 2014. The research was conducted in and around the Metro Vancouver area, and focused mainly on three sources of participants. These three major source locations were the University of British Columbia, Simon Fraser University and GAB youth services in Vancouver's West End. Additional respondents were found through online advertising, which was marginally successful.

The research was able to obtain one hundred and ten completed surveys, which represented a broad cross-section of youth between the ages of 12 and 26, and includes responses from many of the major ethnic and sexual demographic groups represented within Vancouver and who would be relevant to the survey.

The survey itself consisted of two sets of questions; a multiple-choice section and an open-ended question section. The multiple-choice questions were designed to determine the demographic information of the survey participants, and derive no information for the study beyond information about the participants that could be compared to Canadian national demographics. The survey included seven such demographic questions, which included questions on age, ethnic background, sexual orientation and gender identity. The final questions in the multiple-choice section of the survey were related to the athletic lives of the participants. Specifically, the three remaining questions asked about the level of competition the participants were involved in, how long they had participated in athletics and whether they considered themselves out of the closet during their participation.

The majority of the questions on the survey were open-ended and required participants to share and expand on their views regarding numerous topics related to the research. Questions involving the perceptions of participants were considered particularly important, and were used to determine the views of youth about professional and recreational sports and whether there was a consistent belief that these sports organizations were homophobic or transphobic environments. Other questions followed up on queries related to discrimination and asked about the personal experiences of the participants, asking both whether the participants had been victims of discrimination in athletics and also whether homophobic or transphobic discrimination was treated differently than racial or forms of discrimination by coaching or officiating staff. The final questions in the open-ended section related to two possible concepts, which could provide an opportunity for queer youth to participate in athletics or change the underlying culture enough to make athletics more accessible to queer athletes. These questions asked specifically about the willingness of participants to join queer-friendly sports leagues and whether there would be any effect in having more athletes come out of the closet at the professional level.

Important to the research was the need to obtain a sample from different kinds of youth athletes; outreach into the community was successful in finding participants who were involved in a wide variety of sports and also a wide variety of levels of dedication and excellence. This included individuals who had no prior experience in athletics whatsoever to those who participated in elite competitions and represented their regions in official competitions.

While the survey remained open to all members of the public in the target age group, the contents of the survey and the markets to which it was advertised meant that a large oversample of individuals identifying within the queer community were added to the research, relative to their share of the population as noted by Statistics Canada.

Over ninety percent of the surveys were administered through the Internet, allowing the participants to complete the survey at their own pace and ensuring their discretion and privacy in answering these personal questions. The remaining surveys were conducted in person at GAB youth, and were conducted in August as part of a series of unrelated surveys the participants were conducting that day.

Because of the small sample size, definitive conclusions cannot be made about the beliefs of the subject pool. This is particularly true for the sub-groups, some of whom had only a single respondent representing their demographic group. For these situations, the surveys were treated as qualitative surveys and cannot be used to draw conclusions for that group. For the survey as a whole, the margin of error is plus or minus 9.32 percent. This presents difficulties in establishing the views of the population on some of the questions, but is sufficient to determine general trends in the beliefs of the overall youth cohort.

The most important finding to be realized by the research was that youth in the survey still overwhelmingly believe that professional and recreational sports are dominated by homophobia and that there would be significant safety concerns for queer athletes. This perception was found not just in those who identified as part of the queer continuum but also among the heterosexual respondents in the survey; a majority of all demographic groups believed that there was a high level of homophobia in professional sports, and a smaller majority believed that there were high levels of homophobia in either the recreational sports they had participated in themselves, or in the recreational leagues available to them in their communities.

What was interesting to note was that these responses were not similar as respondents continued to engage in athletics. Over three quarters of those who had not participated in athletics believed professional sports to have high levels of homophobia or transphobia, while less than half of survey respondents who had been involved in sports for nine years or more held the same beliefs. However, respondents who had participated in athletics for an extended period of time were more likely than their peers who were not involved to say that homophobia and transphobia in professional sports was dependent on the sport, as opposed to agreeing with blanket statements that all professional sports were intrinsically homophobic or transphobic.

In terms of the views towards recreational sports, most cohorts' perceptions were that there was some measure of homophobia and transphobia in recreational sports, but not nearly as much as in professional sports. The one cohort that disagreed with that assertion was the cohort of participants who had not participated in athletics themselves, with more than half of them believing that recreational sports were highly discriminatory.

Interestingly, the only other group to believe that recreational sports were highly homophobic were those who had participated for more than nine years; all other cohorts had fewer than half their respondents believing that recreational sports were homophobic. While that remains in line with the overall ratio of participants who believed there were high levels of discrimination in recreational athletics, the cohort of non-participants were far more likely to indicate uncertainty about the level of discrimination in sports. Other groups were more likely to volunteer that homophobia was sport or team specific, as opposed to making blanket statements about sports as a whole. Some participants also indicated that it was often just a single individual that were the cause of any discrimination in athletics, suggesting that the problem is not systemic but more interpersonal.

This trend towards greater concern for one's personal safety in sports was also evidenced by the participants' responses to questions about whether they would be exposed to homophobia or transphobia while participating in sports. The trend in this was also positive; in general, those who participated in sports for longer periods of time were less likely to feel concerned about facing discrimination in sports. The cohort of respondents who participated in sports between three and five years were an outlier in this response, with two-thirds of respondents in the cohort expressing some level of concern about facing discrimination in sports.

This cohort of respondents who participated for three to five years was an outlier in all questions relating to their personal concerns and judgments towards sports, and this is likely due to the personal experiences of the members of the cohort. Forty-two percent of respondents in this cohort admitted that they faced some level of discrimination in sport, with half of those respondents noting that the discrimination was sufficient for them to alter their athletic participation rates.

Four participants self-identified as participating in elite leagues during their athletic careers, and their responses to the survey were interesting in comparison to other cohorts, in that they were significantly less optimistic about their experiences compared to the other cohorts. All four mentioned that they were concerned about discrimination and that they had been discriminated against in the course of their athletic career, despite the fact that one is heterosexual and one was not out of the closet during their athletic career.

This compares poorly with other cohorts, which generally displayed fewer concerns about the potential for discrimination in athletics. The research shows that those who participated less or in more casual settings were far less likely to be concerned about the potential for discrimination, with just over half of those who did not participate and those who participated informally stating that the potential for discrimination affected their willingness to participate in athletics

The elite participants were also outliers in the research in that they were one of the few cohorts or demographic groups that is not interested in participating in athletics programs that are designated as queer-friendly or queers-only. Only one of the four elite participants was comfortable or interested in participating in such a league, while nearly three quarters of those who participated informally would be interested in joining such a league.

The responses of the elite participants were interesting in that they suggested that some of the views towards professional sports were in fact correct, based on their assertions of what was done in their own locker rooms, which were a close approximation to the skill level and dedication needed to reach that level of competitiveness as an athlete. The conflicting responses between wanting to stay in mainstream leagues and also fearing discrimination may indicate a concern that the discrimination faced by queer athletes at an elite level is integrated into the sports themselves and is used as a form of motivation to maintain appropriate skill levels.

This dichotomy also appears to hint at the belief that having queer-friendly leagues would preclude the possibility of those leagues being used to develop or maintain high performance athletics in the participants, something that is known to be a concern for athletes who are considering their sport as a profession or college activity. While the elite athletes were fairly negative in their assessment of queer-friendly or queer-only sports leagues, those who participated informally and recreationally were quite supportive of such leagues, with nearly three quarters of informal athletes indicating they would be interested in participating in queer sports leagues, if they were available in their city and had a league for their sport.

Of interest was the fact that those who did not participate at all were also unlikely to be interested in joining a queer-friendly league; fifty-six percent said they would be interested in joining a queer-friendly league, which may be attributed more to a general antipathy towards athletics than anything that was based around discrimination. This view is substantiated by the fact that a similar majority of participants in the cohort stated that the potential for discrimination affected their willingness to participate in athletics.

This seems to lead credence to the belief that queer sports leagues would be something that was seen as a recreational activity where participants would be able to meet with other queer youth in a non-confrontational setting, but for athletes who wished to compete at a higher level these sorts of environments would be detrimental and not appropriate for their development as athletes. This creates an unfortunate choice for athletes in whether they are willing to trade their personal feelings of safety and camaraderie for their ability to grow and become a better player.

It concerns me to read the responses regarding how coaches and other disciplinary staff discussed homophobia and transphobia. Over ninety percent of participants who witnessed or were discriminated against noted that homophobia and transphobia were treated as less severe than racism or other forms of discrimination. While this is a disheartening figure, it remains important to note that more than two-thirds of all participants did not witness any kind of discrimination during their athletics careers.

The trend towards believing in different levels of punishment is strongest in those who were most likely to face persecution and discrimination; those who identified as part of the queer community and were open about their identity were more likely than their heterosexual or closeted peers to believe homophobia and transphobia were likely to result in less punitive measures against perpetrators of discrimination.

Among those who were noted that homophobia and transphobia were treated as less serious by disciplinary staff in their sporting careers, those athletes who were out of the closet were most likely to notice the difference. A forty-four percent plurality of out of the closet athletes claimed that homophobia and transphobia were treated less seriously than racism or other forms of discrimination.

Conversely, only twenty-five percent of participants who identify as heterosexual believed that homophobia or transphobia were treated dissimilarly to any other kind of discrimination. This aligns perfectly with the responses of heterosexual participants, seventy-five percent of whom did not report witnessing or being subjected to homophobia, transphobia or any other kind of discrimination.

In the course of the research, two main ideas came forward as potential solutions to the problem of homophobia and transphobia in sports. The proposed solutions that were commented on by the survey participants were either to have more athletes come out and admit their own sexuality, creating a normalization process in the rest of society and demonstrating through action that queer athletes have the same talents as their heterosexual peers, or to create leagues that were either queer-friendly and had explicit non-discrimination policies or leagues that were queers-only, which would create spaces where only those who identify as part of the queer community would be welcome to participate.

In neither case does the solution apply specifically to the grassroots of athletics where the majority of youth currently participate, and thus the only changes that would be created at these levels would be based on society as a whole being willing to shift their paradigms about what an athlete should and should not be. This is particularly true in the case of having more athletes come out of the closet, as there may be difficulties in creating a connection between professional athletes and a youth in a smaller municipality who is not sure they will succeed at the same level and have that kind of celebrity to protect themselves from discrimination.

The more controversial and potentially more interesting solution was to create leagues that were specifically designated as queer-friendly or queers-only, and which would have specific policies put into place that were meant to protect the safety and identity of queer athletes who participate in those leagues. Like other recreational leagues found in municipalities across North America, each league would be sport specific and would have the potential for different skill levels or tiers to allow for advancement as players became more proficient in their sport.

Most demographic groups were supportive of the idea of queer-friendly leagues, and more than sixty percent of participants agreed that the existence of such a league in their chosen sport would make them more likely to participate in athletics. The results for this question could be divided roughly into two groups; those who identify as part of the societal majority in terms of sexual orientation or gender identity, and those who do not.

Among those who did not identify as heterosexual or cisgendered, the results were nearly unanimous. All but three of the non-heterosexual participants in the research indicated they would be interested or more willing to participate in queer-friendly leagues, including all eight participants who identify as trans, either male to female or female to male. This corresponds with many participants indicating as an optional question that locker rooms and issues regarding the gender binary would serve as additional barriers to participation for queer youth. Because queer-friendly or queers only leagues would have specific policies put into place to address the concerns of sexual minorities, they would provide opportunities to participate without concerns about which gendered changeroom to use in preparation or after completion of the activity.

It was also interesting to note that a majority of those who identified as cisgendered males would also be more likely to participate in athletics if there were queer-friendly sports leagues available in their city. Fifty-five percent of the cisgendered male responses indicated that they would be more interested in playing in queer-friendly leagues. Conversely, among cisgendered participants who declined to state their gender identity, only forty-four percent agreed that they would be more willing to participate if the option of queer-friendly leagues were available to them.

While a strong majority of participants had a greater interest in participating in athletics if they had access to queer-friendly leagues, this trend was not consistent along ethnic lines. First Nations participants were unanimous in their approval and willingness to participate in leagues such as these, but only one third of South Asians were similarly interested. The sole participant of Middle Eastern descent also disagreed strongly with the concept of having queer-friendly leagues. In addition, only half of participants of Asian ancestry would have been more willing to participate in athletics in queer-friendly leagues.

This is not to say that it was solely Caucasians who were interested in participating in queer-friendly leagues. Only sixty-two percent of Caucasian participants indicated they would be more likely to participate in sports if they had access to queer-friendly sports leagues, with one in seven Caucasian participants being unsure of how their participation rates would change if given the opportunity to participate. Strong support for queer-friendly leagues was also found among Hispanic participants, with two- thirds of them indicating they would be more likely to participate in athletics within queer-friendly leagues.

One of the major concerns raised about queer-friendly leagues was that they would fail to be fully inclusive of those who do not identify as part of the queer continuum, and thus would not provide a welcoming space for heterosexual or cisgendered athletes who consider themselves allies of queer rights and queer athletes. Four of the participants volunteered without prompting that they were concerned that queer-friendly leagues would create a sense of segregation and discrimination between different kinds of leagues, with several other participants indicating that all leagues should be queer-friendly instead of having to create new leagues to achieve that same purpose.

With regards to the research itself, the vast majority of participants in the research indicated that having more out queer athletes would help reduce discrimination in both professional and recreational sports. One hundred and four of the one hundred and ten participants agreed with this statement, while only three participants disagreed with the idea that having more queer athletes would provide meaningful benefits to reducing homophobia and transphobia in athletics. The near unanimity of the results from the survey indicate that this kind of act would be of great importance to the grassroots and should not be discounted as a means of creating change in the local organizations that cater to youth athletics.

While every demographic group and division of participants in the study was nearly unanimous in their belief that having more athletes come out would be a positive step towards reducing homophobia and transphobia in sports, the results were not entirely uniform. Those who had not participated in sports at all were the least likely to believe that having more out athletes would be successful in reducing homophobia. Two of the three participants who believed having professional athletes come out of the closet would not reduce discrimination were participants who stated they had not participated in athletics themselves.

Those who did not identify as part of the gender identity spectrum were also less likely than their peers to believe that having more out athletes would lead to a reduction in discrimination in athletics, with one third of the participants in this demographic indicating that they either disagreed with the premise of the question or were unsure of the effects that professional athletes coming out would have on youth sports.

The only other group to register notable levels of disapproval of the premise of the question were those participants who identified as cisgendered without identifying the gender they identify with. These participants were simply unsure of what the resulting impact and consequences would be, and were not willing to agree or disagree with the belief that professional athletes coming out would reduce homophobia or transphobia in youth sports.

The two groups that were least likely to agree with the idea of out athletes also had very different potential reasons for their opposition or concern. For those who identified as cisgendered and were unsure of the results of coming out, this is something I believe can be attributed to the fact that it is not a concern for those individuals; these are people who are part of the societal majority in that they identify with their biological sex. Both participants were also part of ethnic groups that compose large segments of the population in Vancouver; for these individuals, they are less likely to be able to appreciate the impact athletes coming out would have on queer youth because they are simply not part of that demographic group. For these individuals, it's a non-issue, which is a positive sign of greater acceptance in itself, and it also shows that it is unlikely that queer youth will face a backlash when they come out.

For those who do not identify as part of the gender identity spectrum at all, their reasoning for being sceptical is likely to be somewhat different. These are individuals who are not part of the societal majority, and even among the minority of the queer community they are a distinct minority. Because of their position in society as part of a very small minority, they may have greater difficulty identifying and associating with the gains that have been made by the queer community over the past few decades in terms of their legal rights. This is similar to other current concerns within the queer community in which members of the transgender community often feel as though their issues are not brought to the forefront in order to fight for the goals of cisgendered members of the queer community, who are able to use their numerical superiority to control the agenda. In this case, a majority of those participants who do not identify as part of the gender identity spectrum were still supportive of the idea that having more queer athletes would reduce discrimination, but because they are so deep in the minority themselves, they may not see how decreasing homophobia or transphobia would translate into greater understanding and support of their own position in society.

Both solutions presented by the research and commented upon by participants are viable and are likely to have a positive effect on reducing homophobia and transphobia in sports. As solutions, they are primary steps that need to be taken in order to create positive athletic environments for all youth. What neither solution does is provide immediate pressure on currently existing leagues to change their policies and practices to create safe environments, something that was highlighted by many of the participants of the survey.

What these potential solutions do provide is an opportunity for queer youth to become involved in athletics while policymakers craft a more durable solution to the problem of homophobia and transphobia in athletics. Vancouver has been a leader in the creation of these sorts of leagues, showing that there is a strong market for these kinds of activities and that youth will participate if they have an opportunity to do. According to the Vancouver group Queer Active there are seventeen different sports organizations that are either queer-friendly or are entirely composed of members of the queer community. Many of these organizations have partnerships or agreements with the City of Vancouver and are able to use city facilities in the same manner as traditional youth sports leagues.

The major benefit of these potential solutions is that they are easy to implement into the current athletic culture of a city; the main obstacle to the creation of such leagues is the concern that there will be insufficient members to participate and fund the league's operations. This research shows that there is strong interest in athletic participation and would likely be replicable in other locations.

With regards to creating queer-friendly leagues, the solution itself does provide opportunities for queer youth and their allies to have a safe space to engage in athletics without having to fear discrimination from other players or coaches, but it also creates a form of self-segregation that would seem to run counter to the idea of full integration in society. These sports leagues would have a strong, stable membership based on the findings of the research, but they would also do very little to effect change in other organizations. One potential response from current sports organizations would be to simply do nothing, knowing that if any of their current members were feeling unsafe in their current league, those youth could simply transfer and play in these new queer-friendly leagues.

The segregation into queer and 'mainstream' leagues would also create a potentially harmful situation for athletes who have not come out of the closet, which included thirty-four percent of the research population. For these individuals who have not admitted to others that they were part of the queer community, joining one of these leagues may be seen as a tacit admission of their divergent sexual orientation or gender identity and thus could present concerns for athletes being outed before they were ready to confront their peers with the information. In such situations, rather than creating safer environments for younger queer individuals to participate in sports, the segregated leagues would have the opposite effect and make youth more likely to face ridicule and discrimination.

The effects of having more professional athletes come out of the closet is a bit more difficult to determine in terms of its effect on the grassroots organizations in North America, though recent evidence serves to suggest that it has a neutral effect on societal homophobia at worst, and at best it is helping to eliminate discrimination in professional athletics. Most noticeably, the effect on having more athletes admit their sexuality has been causing greater numbers of other athletes to publicly come out, with the effect being amplified most at the collegiate level[vii].

The media coverage surrounding Michael Sam is the most obvious recent example, but in the last year a number of collegiate athletes with potential professional careers have started to come out to their teams and the media without facing backlash[viii]. In many cases, when interviewed by media about why they chose to come out, athletes are reporting that it was because other queer athletes came out and reported little opposition to their coming out that served as the final reason to come out themselves[ix].

However, while the effect on college athletes has been promising, there has been a limited impact on professional sports thus far, and the effect on local sporting organizations is unknown. This would seem to indicate that while there is overall support for the concept of creating safe spaces in athletics for queer individuals, the professional leagues themselves have fully adjusted to the concept. This is disappointing because many professional teams have made conscious efforts to target queer consumers as part of their marketing schemes, including many 'gay days' for their teams, but those same teams are still either defending discriminatory athletes on their teams or refusing to partner with outside organizations to make athletics safer for queer athletes[x].

It is this safety component and the views of other players and the leagues that is the most likely reason why queer athletes at the professional level are not coming out. In the world of professional athletics, it's become necessary to ensure that players remain as popular as possible in order to increase sales for the team ownership and management. Creating controversy detracts from this, and it appears that sports team owners still believe that homosexual players would cause a controversy that would be a distraction for the team.

For players themselves, there is also the concern that they will become unsupported and that their careers will be damaged if they come out, which is part of where outside organizations must intervene to demonstrate the appeal of having queer athletes involved in sports. Programs like the 'You Can Play' project are vital to demonstrating to professional athletes that there are networks available that would help if a professional athlete was to come out[xi]. These partnerships are still in their infancy, but they must begin to show that they are accomplishing their objectives before professional athletes determine that it is not in their personal interest to come out and serve as positive role models for queer athletes.

Because of this lack of support for professional athletes, young queer athletes are lacking role models in the professional athletic world that they can look up to and believe they can emulate in the future. Having these college athletes come out is a good first step, and there's no doubt that doing so helps provide comfort to queer athletes who hear about these coming out stories. The fact remains that college athletes do not get as much media attention as professional athletes, and that there are far more college athletes than professional athletes. Thus for many queer youth, college athletics is seen as insufficient; it's a good starting place but it's not where queer athletes want to be, and until they begin to see paid athletes coming out they will lack the courage to come out themselves.

The impact of professionals coming out should be noticeable for queer youth almost immediately; by providing these role models in an area of life that the youth are interested in, it shows that societal acceptance is possible and that being queer is not a barrier to participating in athletics. Beyond assuaging doubts about the ability to participate in athletics as a queer individual, it also would provide an opportunity to demonstrate greater societal acceptance for homosexuality and transsexuality by having these athletes be positively received by their teammates and wider athletics world.

On a local level, having these professional athletes come out without facing discrimination or abuse would force local leagues to accept that there are queer athletes and that some of their own members could possibly be part of the queer community. This could potentially create a space for dialogue on the need for new policies regarding discrimination and how to teach young athletes about diversity in their workplace, as the athletics world at a professional level is considered a workplace for the athletes.

This would be especially true for many organizations that partner with professional sports teams to provide additional mentoring and coaching to their students. Many professional sports teams send their players to help mentor and coach local organizations in their area, one of the major examples being the Toronto Blue Jays, whose alumni organization spends countless hours working with youth in order to teach baseball skills to youth in leagues throughout Canada[xii]. Having organizations work with an openly gay athlete would give the organizations and their players a chance to see that the player him or herself is no different than when they were closeted, which will help foster greater tolerance and understanding about the issues facing queer athletes.

Athletics continues to be one of the few places left in society that is consistently believed to be considered hostile to the rights of queer individuals. This will change over time, especially as more athletes come out and celebrate who they are. While we are working towards a day of total acceptance for queer individuals in society, we can still do much to hasten towards that day. The most important way to accomplish this is to change the way sports are perceived, and to ensure that there remains a consistent force opposing discrimination and focusing on creating spaces where queer athletes can be celebrated for their achievements in their sport.

What has been learned is that there is a desire on the part of queer youth to be involved, that they want to be part of sports and athletics like their heterosexual peers, but they are continually turning away from healthier lifestyles because of overriding concerns that they will not be welcome among their peers if they choose to participate in sports. As this happens, there remains an increasing number of athletes who are coming out, but are not being recognized by the media for their actions, furthering the belief that sports and homosexuality cannot mix and that one has to choose between those two aspects of their identity. Breaking down these barriers and allowing individuals to realize that they can be both a queer person and an athlete is the key to ending discrimination in sport.

The reasons for wanting to have higher engagement in athletics could not be more clear; those who engage in athletic endeavours, even at a recreational level, report better physical health and higher health outcomes because of their physical activities, and playing as part of a team provides another social connection for queer youth. These connections can reduce the likelihood of mental and emotional disorders, and can also be seen as a means of connecting queer youth to their communities. With queer youth being far more likely than their heterosexual peers to report emotional and psychological problems, providing an additional support network and means of relieving stress should remain a top priority for policymakers in the near future.

As a closeted gay male, participating in athletics was a conflicted time in my life. On the one hand, I genuinely enjoyed participating in sports, especially on the competitive teams where I had made myself at home and was succeeding with. On the other hand, it was difficult to be around my teenage teammates who were constantly talking about their girlfriends and their personal lives and who were also picking on me somewhat regularly because I wasn't part of those conversations. They knew I was different and not really from the same group as them, but they weren't entirely sure how. Being teenagers, this eventually meant that comments were raised suggesting that I was gay, and because I was unwilling to lie and deny those accusations, it become commonplace for my teammates to talk about my being gay and making derogatory statements about me because of it.

Having said that, I never found sports at any level to be explicitly homophobic or discriminatory towards anyone. Unfortunate comments were made and they shouldn't be tolerated because of the harm that could be caused by those statements, but the truth of the matter is that we were kids and we were acting like kids. Even when I was being treated badly by my teammates and ostracized for the possibility of being gay, I never felt like I was a total outsider on the team. It's important to note that I did not become active in athletics in order to find a social network or group of friends; I had a strong circle of friends outside of my athletic endeavours, and as a rule I did not actually spend my leisure time with my teammates outside of when we were at practices or games together. This meant that in many ways, I became an outsider to the team by choice, as I didn't choose to spend more time with them when I had the opportunity, and they weren't particularly eager to have me join them. This was never about my homosexuality, either before or after I came out, and was based more on the different personalities we had and how I did not understand them on a cultural level. Which isn't to say that I didn't bond with my team, we spent a lot of time together on road trips getting to know each other better and gelling as a team.

What I saw from sports as a relatively competitive athlete was that once the game was on and we were actually expected to perform, my teammates and the opposition were incredibly focused on the sport itself, and anything that took away or distracted from the game at hand was considered unacceptable and not worth discussing at that point in time. For me, this meant that even if they didn't consider me a personal friend of theirs, my teammates were always willing to respect me because they could see my talent on the field and understand that I was a contributing member of the team. This helped more in my baseball career when I was one of the better players on my team and was able to take on a leadership role on the field instead of having to worry that the common stereotype of gays men being poor at sports would be applied to me and would serve as a means of my teammates discriminating against me or becoming abusive towards me.

After coming out, I found that my sexual orientation became a non-issue with my teammates unless I made it one by being inappropriate or otherwise highlighting the fact that I had a different sexual orientation than the rest of the team. Most were quite happy to continue treating me the way they had before, with the notable exception of being more conscious of what they said with regards to comments that could be perceived as homophobic. This did not actually continue on very long, and like most teenagers my teammates started reverting back and using terms that could be considered homophobic around me. This didn't bother me as much since I knew they were not meaning it as an attack on me and was simply how they spoke and how they bonded as a team.

Beyond the way that some of my teammates treated me after coming out, there wasn't all that much that changed for me as an athlete. I still competed just as much as I had before, and the ability to separate my personal life from my athletic life was genuinely appreciated by everyone, especially since as teenagers many of them were not interested in hearing from someone lecturing about the need for equal rights. They were interested and on a personal level they supported the idea of equality, but on the sports fields they felt that we already were equal, and that it didn't need to be re-litigated through a lecture or pleas for understanding and compassion; I would be judged solely on what I did as a player and that was incredibly liberating as a queer player who had just come out of the closet. Actually, I found that my teammates respected me more because of what I did and how I came out, and the resulting improvement in my play helped mask any concerns they may have had about my sexual orientation or any discomfort they may have had. I was glad to find that after coming out I was still just as welcome at team events as I had always been.

The leagues themselves weren't all that interested in worrying about my sexual orientation either; I was a player and I was in good standing, that was all that mattered as far as they were concerned. Most didn't even know I was gay even after I came out, and that suited most of them perfectly well, and it suited me as well. Improving my game play helped get me more attention from the coaches, but for the most part nothing really changed in terms of how I was treated. There also wasn't much done that would be perceived as push back against the way homophobic or transphobic comments were addressed on the team either, the coaches and other adults present seemed to believe that the comments could be dealt with without their intervention, and that in itself actually made me feel better about the situation. I suppose from the perspective of being good allies they probably should have intervened on my behalf and stated that they were opposed to that kind of language, but doing so would have made it more difficult for me to grow comfortable with myself and would have made the team more tense, so it was left to me to defend myself in a way that would promote professionalism amongst the players, which I found to be refreshing, even if it would be different from how most people would expect a queer player to want their coach to react.

My coming out journey was in many respects similar to most athletes, and in some ways is not yet complete, nor will it ever truly be complete. The first thing I decided to do when coming out to people was accept that it was part of who I was, but that I would not let it dominate who I was as a person. To that end, I generally do not tell people that I'm gay, and instead just talk about my life and let people draw their own conclusions about what my sexual orientation is. I feel that in doing so I'm not hiding myself from the world, but I'm also expressing that I think of it as a non-issue as far as my life goes and that it should be considered a non-issue when interacting with me as well.

From a young age I realized that I was different from my peers and that in many cases I was attracted to them physically. This realization came as I was entering puberty and coming close to graduating from elementary school. By this time I had already become fully immersed in the athletic world, having played hockey and baseball for a number of years in my community. Outside of my two major sports of hockey and baseball, I also was involved with my elementary school volleyball team and joined a community basketball team. When I was ready to start coming out when I was fourteen, I had already quit hockey, volleyball and basketball, but had joined a local curling club and was beginning to experience success as a curler. I was also experiencing varying levels of success in my baseball career, having started to consistently make the cut for the all star team in my hometown and developing as a pitcher.

It was clear to me at this point that I was secure in my place as an athlete, but I was having difficulty reconciling my athleticism and the stereotype of gay people that I had seen in the media of men who were both incapable and uninterested in athletics. This internal conflict often led me to being quite ill, such that my athletics careers were not as good as they could have been had I been healthier and better able to compete on a regular basis. In my early years as a junior curler, I was deep in the closet and actually started dating a female teammate so as to better provide cover for myself and avoid the scrutiny of those who may have been watching me. It is a popular belief that football or baseball has the most homophobic environment, but my belief at the time was that curling was comprised of largely conservative individuals who would not tolerate someone so different from themselves, so I pursued the relationship as a means of making everyone assume I was straight as well.

This didn't work for me; I found that I was conflicted about everything that was happening around me and it felt wrong to continually hide such an important part of myself from the people who I was supposed to be bonding with in order to achieve our mutual goals of athletic success. As it was, I had already been outed to my family by an accident, so I already knew that my parents would support me regardless of who I was or what I did. That made things easier to come out to my team, since I had already done the hard part of becoming out to my family.

I decided that it would be easier to come out to my teammates one at a time, and also that it would be best to do so during the off season, which would give us all time apart if we found that things became awkward between us. My usual means of coming out to someone involved a round of golf; we were all baseball players, but most of my teammates also enjoyed playing golf, so I found it was easier to go and take them with me to the pitch and putt and get a round in before dropping the news on them. I should note that I played terribly in those rounds, which I partially attribute to my nerves about coming out to someone, but also because I'm a lousy golfer.

The first person I came out to on the team was the coach's son and my usual catcher. He had gone to a private school and was one of the people most vocal in questioning me about my sexuality, so I was not sure how he would react when I told him. We also had a bit of a personal rivalry between us; we had played for opposing teams as younger children and we were both talented players, so we found that we were often opponents on separate all star teams. This rivalry got personal at many points, with him attacking me over my perceived sexual orientation and me responding in kind about his weight issues, neither of which would be considered acceptable now and in hindsight were not acceptable then either.

We were actually just heading back towards the clubhouse when I did come out. We had been getting to the point where we were devolving into our usual insults and generally rude behaviour, except this time I did not join in the banter and attacking. Instead, I got really quiet and I just said to stop, that I was gay and that he was crossing a line. The results were satisfying; I can truthfully say that before that point, I hadn't seen anyone actually go slack jawed in front of me, and to see it in real life and not just as an animated cartoon was a bit of a gift. I think that he, like most people, thought that because I was something of a jock and did play sports as well as I did, that I couldn't be gay and anything that he and others said were just insults that wouldn't have any meaning to me.

Those initial few seconds where he wasn't able to articulate a response were absolutely terrifying; I had no idea how he was going to eventually react, and instinctively I believed that the very worst was coming and that I would be forced to defend myself against a teammate. It came as a relief to me when he regained the ability to speak and he apologized for all the things he had said over the past few years that we had been playing together. I don't know if I meant it then, but I accepted his apology and explained that I did understand why he and others talked the way he did, and he in turn said that he would try and watch what he says a bit more closely. We actually spent the rest of the afternoon just talking about what it would mean for the team and what it meant for me as a person, as it turned out he had a lot of questions for me that I tried to answer as best I could. The next season he kept his word and he did try to keep a lid on things, not just with himself but also with some of the other members of the team, which gave me the courage I needed to start coming out to the rest of them over the next season.

I did eventually come out to at least part of my curling team, which I found to be more difficult simply because we were a closer community and that there were only the four of us. Having only four team members meant that we had to trust each other and not have any kind of personality conflict, since it would be difficult for the rest of the team to address those concerns if there were any between two players. I found that telling my curling teammates was easier when we were in the middle of a game or practice and their focus wasn't entirely on what I was saying; most of them simply acknowledged it and carried on with what we were doing, and most weren't entirely sure why I bothered to tell them, since it wasn't really their business. Once again, this was on a competitive team and we decided collectively that we had other things we needed to worry about instead of each other's personal lives.

Prior to coming out in both my full time sports, I found that I was very cautious and conflicted on what my role on each team would be. I very often remained quiet during team meetings or any other conference that was just for the team players, preferring instead to try and blend in and not get noticed for fear of facing more homophobic commentary from my teammates. This extended to how I played on the field and the ice. I tried to keep my distance emotionally from my teammates and was more reserved that I should be as a player. Instead of allowing the emotions of the game to take over and to feel the adrenaline of the game, I was spending more time thinking about what would happen if they all knew my secret. As those kinds of thoughts became more prevalent in my mind, my abilities began to suffer and I started to become a drag on my teams.

This came as a shock to me as I had always been one of the better players on my teams, and to start being a drain on our ability to win games and stay in contention for the league finals was something that I found intolerable. It was also beginning to strain my relationships with my teammates who sensed that something was wrong but they were not able to determine what my problem was. I never considered quitting, I love sports too much to have contemplating giving it up entirely, but I was seriously concerned that I was hurting my teams by dealing with this internal conflict between being gay and being an athlete, and I realized that I would have to start telling my teammates in order to fix the problem in my game.

More than anything, I was just distracted and put in a position where I was not only unable to play at my best, but given the positions I would regularly play in with my baseball team, I was put in situations that could be dangerous to me. This, combined with my own natural fear of being hit with a ball, meant I was even less able to play at the calibre that was expected of me. Instead of charging towards the ball in order to make a good play, I found my first instinct was to step back in order to give myself more time to react, instead of trusting my abilities and my reflexes to ensure that I wasn't harmed and anticipated the bounce a ball would take. As can be imagined, this didn't work nearly as well as I had thought; I started making mistakes on the bounce the ball would take and missing my plays badly. More than just missing and causing my team to suffer, I started getting bit by the ball a fair bit more because I was often off-balance and unable to react properly once the ball did take an unexpected bounce. So for all the efforts I did to try and distract myself from my internal conflict of whether to come out or not, all it did was exacerbate the problems I already had on the field and it didn't do anything to help me decide whether to come out or not.

It sounds cliche and in many ways it is, but after I started coming out I was a different person among my teammates. I started taking on a leadership position on my baseball team and earning the grudging respect of my teammates, including some who disliked me on a personal level and would prefer to see me fail. This came mainly through the fact that once the game was on and we were focused on the sport, they knew they could count on me to be one of their top players again. My pitching became far better once I came out to my catcher, and we started trusting each other far more. I started posting wins as a pitcher and the team started pulling out of the slump we had been in the previous year. It's a deep secret of mine, but for all the years I played baseball I was actually terrified of the ball hitting me and being seriously injured by it. I still am, which is part of why I retired from baseball after high school, but I found that after coming out and dealing with that kind of fear of being rejected by my teammates, the ball itself wasn't as frightening as it used to be. I started making more and better plays, and even my batting average started going up once I was more comfortable around the team.

As for curling, I was always in a leadership position on the teams I played for there, but I was also very concerned about maintaining my position and I was very guarded among my teammates to ensure that I was always in charge. Part of that was being young, but a lot of it was attributed to the fact that I needed to be in control so that no one knew I was gay and thought less of me for it. Once I was out and didn't have to worry about how my teammates thought of me, I was able to assert leadership without having to be so jealous of other members of my team, and I found I could relax a lot more around them. My teammates continued to change and coming out to my new teammates was easier because of my past experiences. Most of my final junior teammates were quite excited about having a gay teammate, and we talked a fair bit about the stereotypes and turned it into a bit of a running joke that I defied nearly all those stereotypes.

Curling also produced the most interesting response to my being gay, and I don't entirely know if it was because I was a gay teammate or whether this was just a sign of insanity among my teammates. Each year the team had to think about what our uniform would look like, and as this was a new team we needed new jackets and shirts for everyone. We decided pretty easily on jackets that were representative of our club and had their traditional colours, but we weren't sure what to do for shirts, which were supposed to be worn by all members of the team. Someone on the team who wasn't me suggested that we wear pink shirts as a way of differentiating ourselves from everyone else. Pink being a colour that was associated with the queer community, I found it quite interesting that my teammates were so eager to take on the colour. Everyone seemed excited about it as well, which I found quite surprising. These were the same teammates that I enjoyed the long running joke with, so it made sense on a certain level, but it was still quite surprising to have that level of implied support.

While as a team we weren't as successful in my later junior years of curling, I did find that I was personally able to curl with more confidence in my abilities and my teammates, and that in turn made me a better player. My confidence in my own abilities grew and I started calling and making more difficult shots. This in turn garnered the attention of those who were watching me and did help ensure that I would have a place in the men's league. My abilities also gained the respect of my opponents who were surprised to see me play with the confidence I had at the age I was at.

Those years that I was out to my curling teammates were some of my best years playing, we were successful in almost all our endeavours and I actually was selected to play on a men's team while retaining junior league eligibility. I improved my skills and won a few awards for my skills. I also got to know my teammates far better than I otherwise would, and count myself lucky that I still talk with a couple of them every so often, even though it's been years since we all played together.

I'm the first to admit that coming out to teammates is a challenge and it's more than a little terrifying. You spend most of your free time with these people, and you have to trust them on at least some level in order to mesh as a team. The fear of rejection is incredibly strong once you have those bonds in place, and they can make it nearly impossible to want to put yourself in a position where those bonds are strained are broken. This is especially true for younger people or those who use sports as one of their primary means of finding new friends to add to their social circle; losing that access to sports or fearing that loss of access because of a bad reaction to your coming out can be especially hurtful. For many people who come out, this fear can be almost unbearable and it leads to those people being closeted for most of their lives.

The first thing to do is probably the most important, and that's to breathe. Seriously, psyching yourself out and making the issue bigger than it needs to be is not going to help you. Which isn't to say that it's not important; coming out to people is one of the most important things you can do and it puts you in an incredibly vulnerable position. For the person or people you're coming out to though, it's very likely going to come as a complete shock, and if you're already feeling tense or nervous about the encounter they're going to pick up on that and start becoming more tense and nervous themselves. All that is going to do is make everything much worse than it needs to be and will likely make either you or the other person blow things out of proportion. Staying calm and in control of your nerves is going to help show the person you're coming out to that it doesn't have to be a big deal or a massive change in your relationship, it's just you opening up about yourself a bit more and telling them something about your personal life that they may not have known before.

You know your teammates better than most other people will, so it is up to you to determine whether you should be meeting with them as a group or if coming out to them individually is better. However you choose to do so, picking an appropriate time to do so is very important, particularly when playing on competitive teams. Appropriate times are going to be in situations where telling people and potentially putting them in a conflicted head space is not going to put them in physical danger or compromise their own ability to enjoy the sport you're participating in. Generally this means waiting until after games are over or the season as a whole is over, depending on the kind of team you're on and how much you trust the people around you to react positively to the news of your coming out. Some people, however, wait until the beginning of the next season to tell people, especially when they're expecting either to be on a new team themselves or that their old team will have a number of new recruits added to it. By waiting until the new season begins, it gives your teammates an opportunity to decide if they are going to feel comfortable around you before they have committed themselves to the team.

In terms of actually telling people, it helps just to be very blunt about it and not dance around the issue. More than anything this is to help with your own nerves, if you're continually going to be dancing and creeping up on the issue it generally makes you more nervous and concerned about how your teammate will react. Explaining to the person how important this is to you and that you are telling them because you trust them and want them to understand you better is also quite helpful, as it puts the other person at ease and gets them to understand that it's not that you're trying to burden them with a secret that needs to be kept. The important thing is to continue to be as calm as possible under the circumstances and try to keep control of the conversation.

Beyond the actual act of coming out to the other person, there's always going to be that aftermath where the other person responds and starts taking their own place in the conversation. For athletes that are coming out to their teammates, this is a stressful time and can also be an aggravating time when you may have to deal with potential stereotypes that your teammates are going to throw at you. For the most part, your teammates don't mean this in a malicious sense; it's just what society has generally accepted as a stereotype of gay athletes, and that may mean that you have to answer a lot of awkward or peculiar questions and dispel some myths about queer individuals. It's not meant to be a personal attack, but it often can feel that way when you're answering those same questions over and over again. Be prepared for your teammates to be as forthright with you as you were with them when you came out to them; most people will assume that if you are going to be as candid as it takes to come out to someone that they also have permission to respond with an equal level of candor. Once again, this is not meant specifically to harm you or otherwise frustrate you, it's just a response that your teammate is having and may be based on the shock to their system by upsetting the stereotypes they may have believed in.

When I came out to my catcher, I thought it was going to be something that I instantly regretted, simply because of his background and how much he was involved in talking down to me about my perceived sexual orientation in the past. It was actually really interesting to see how much he changed and how quickly it happened. Obviously there were a lot of questions and he wanted me to answer them as much as possible, but the questions themselves were never all that invasive and were certainly not meant to harm me or ridicule me. For the most part they were just questions about how it all works and just addressing some of the stereotypes. I think for my own part, staying calm and realising that it was just meant to be questions and genuinely needing the information meant that he was able to stay calm and not panic either. It really did make the whole situation far better than it could have been, even if some of the questions were a bit bizarre. My other teammates were even better, at least with regards to having questions for me. Most of them just accepted it without much thought or comment, and for the most part I was just confirming things they had already been thinking were true about me. The wide range of responses that I got showed me that it's important to prepare for anything when you're planning on coming out to people, but for the most part the people you come out to are going to be accepting of who you are and happy that you're able to trust them enough to tell them the truth.

Hopefully this doesn't happen, but should you encounter a scenario where your teammate responds poorly to you coming out, make sure you leave yourself with a way to leave the situation safely. Once you're away from the situation, take a few minutes to relax and gain control of yourself, being initially rejected when coming out can leave people very tense and scared. This is all natural, but it shouldn't completely dominate your thoughts. It's important that you not give up on that person either, many people will initially react poorly because of past beliefs or reasons that are outside your control. Sometimes it really is just that the shock of the information you've given the person is too much for them to process and they react poorly because of it. Those people will get over it as time goes on and they will see that you're still the same person you were before and will start becoming more of an ally once they've had an opportunity to process it themselves. Even those who are initially unsupportive are likely to at least respect you in public if the rest of your team is supportive. It hurts to hear, but it makes an impact on people who reject you to see that you don't let them frustrate you or force you back in the closet; they may have reasons outside your control or understanding to react poorly, but it's been proven in research done around the world that actually knowing queer people and interacting with them helps create more tolerant individuals as they learn that their stereotypes and assumptions aren't true and that you aren't any different than you were before.

Whether you come out to a large group or just an individual, the only thing you can really worry about is yourself and your own reactions to the situation. Keeping calm and in control of yourself is of vital importance, as well as ensuring that you have an opportunity to defuse any situation that may arise from you coming out to your teammates or coaches. Queer rights are gaining acceptance throughout the world and more people than ever are seeing that we're no different than our heterosexual peers and neighbours. We live in the most accepting society for queer people that's existed in the Western world yet and even children are being exposed to more positive queer role models in the school. Coming out is still scary and terrifying, especially in the final frontier of homophobia, but even sports are becoming more accepting. We have gay days at our sports events and more professionals than ever are coming out, so keep those things in mind when and if you decide to come out to your teammates, there will be groups and people ready to support you. Those people are going to include your teammates, so don't be afraid of letting them know who you are and how you coming out benefits the team.

Once you're already through the process of coming out and telling your team that you are an openly queer person, the hard part of actually ensuring that you're able to continue contributing to the team starts up. Your teammates and coaches are going to be watching you pretty carefully in the immediate aftermath of you coming out, checking to make sure that you are actually okay and that coming out hasn't been about anything other than ensuring you can perform at the best of your abilities. Sometimes, it's going to be going through the minds of your teammates or coaches that you came out as a kind of stunt in order to gauge people's reactions or to get some kind of differential treatment. While this is a silly notion on the face of it, some people will think that way and it's important to show that it's not about getting everyone talking about you. Besides, there are a lot of other things that a team should be talking about with regards to one of their players instead of talking about who they're attracted to, it shouldn't be an issue and it wouldn't come up at all except that you as a player feel the need to be completely honest with yourself and others. So just keep in mind for yourself that you haven't changed, but the way some people are going to perceive you and interact with you will change, and that it shouldn't be considered personal or meant to slight you. They may just be wanting to ensure that you are still able to play your best and improve as a player, which should be the most important thing for all members of the team.

I didn't play in sports that required a locker room or required that you change in each other's presence. When we would finish our baseball games we'd almost always travel home or to the hotel in our uniforms and just change once we got home and could be assured of a hot shower to work the soreness out of our muscles and a hearty meal to replenish the nutrients we needed to keep doing this day after day. It was a similar situation with curling, but even more pronounced as we weren't even potentially covered in dirt or other debris from the field; all we did was play on the ice. Though in both sports we had specific uniforms that we wore and were expected of us once we were in game, most or all of it could be worn at home and on the trip to the game location. Locker rooms and changing are thus concepts that are not familiar to me as a competitive athlete, but there are certain principles that are pretty self-evident and should be followed by all people in general that need to be reiterated for queer athletes, particularly after you come out to your team.

This is really obvious but has to be said; don't stare or make other teammates feel as though you're checking them out or otherwise making them feel objectified. To be blunt, it's not what you're supposed to be there for and it's not what your teammates are there for, even if some of them are queer as well. Playing team sports should be about making friends and for the love of the game, sometimes even for the competitiveness of the game if you're more interested in competitive athletics. Your teammates aren't meant to be your eye candy, and doing so really puts a strain on teammates who find it harder to trust you because they're not sure what your intentions towards them are anymore. For teenagers and other youth athletes in particular, making sure your teammates don't think you're checking them out is important because of how volatile emotions can be; the last thing anyone wants is to start a fight over something that's not even actually happening, and unfortunately that means care is needed to ensure there aren't any misunderstandings by anyone.

Stand up for yourself. You're all on the same team and are supposed to be working together to get better at your sport. No one needs to be ridiculed by their teammates because of who they are, and that's something that you don't have to put up with even if you're in the closet. I strongly believe that athletics should be teaching people leadership skills as well as sports skills, and that can start by something as simple as calling out people for discriminatory words and actions on the field. It doesn't need to be an angry attack on the person, something as simple as saying that it's not cool to be putting people down and to be a better person than that can be enough, and it shows that you're willing to stand by your teammates when they need it, instead of doing the easy thing and ignoring it or joining in to be part of the crowd. If you are out when this happens, then feel free to talk about how that affects you personally and that you're not going to put up with abuse from your teammates. Baseball was definitely the harder sport for me to stay involved with after coming out, simply because of how many people were on the team and how wide ranging the views were towards my being out. There were still a few guys that would throw comments my way and the only thing I had to do was remind them that they were all talk, and that I was still on the team and deserving of their respect. If they had a problem with that, they could take it up with someone who cared and see how it went because the rest of the team had moved on and did not care, so it was time for them to do the same. It usually worked and certainly meant that people were less willing to show opposition after I finished telling them that they needed to grow up

More than anything, just don't let anything become a big deal now that you're out or are thinking of coming out. It's going to hurt when you hear your teammates say things that could be perceived as homophobic or transphobic, or when they're directly insulting you or giving you grief for who you are. Blowing up or giving them a reaction other than your professionalism or disapproval for their immature tactics is just going to make you more frustrated and put you off your game, which is probably part of what they are trying to do anyway. That isn't to say you should just ignore them and let people say what they want about you, but it doesn't have to devolve into a brawl or a shouting match between teammates. Going through your usual routine and not paying any undue attention to disappointing reactions to coming out will do more to end the bullying behaviour than playing into their stereotypes or actions and engaging on their level; at some point the rest of your team and the coaching staff with decide it's gone too far and intervene for you. As much as it may hurt, the one thing that you shouldn't want to be doing is to complain to the coaches or to other players about it. There may well be policies that are meant to protect you, and reminding them of those policies yourself can sometimes be a good deterrent, but getting the coaching staff involved should be a last resort, as it shows that you're being severely affected by the bullying behaviour and that you're also not able to address the problem without help. That may be a short term solution, and it will likely stop the behaviour for a little while, but once the other player feels that they're able to do so again they'll start up the bullying behaviour and they will likely escalate because they know you're not able to respond effectively, except to tell someone else.

Should issues persist over time and some of your teammates prove unwilling or unable to remain professional with you, talk to the person one on one and try to figure out what it is that's bothering them about you being out, and how it didn't bother them to have you on the team before they knew that you identified as part of the queer community. It may be that your teammate is having difficulty reconciling their personal beliefs with what they know of you, and that it is causing them a similar kind of personal conflict that you likely had when you were first deciding whether to come out or not. This is particularly true for people who may have grown up with strong religious beliefs that characterized homosexuality in a negative light, and thus knowing you provides a contrast between what they had been told about homosexuality and what they already know of you as a person. The kinds of stereotypes that people grow up with and spend their whole lives hearing are the most difficult to break, and when they're based on minority groups that are not obvious to society it can be harder still to break them because there's no obvious counterpoint that people can look at to serve as a way of discounting those stereotypes. By coming out and providing that counterpoint, you are forcing people to confront things they have otherwise accepted as a universal truth, and that's going to mean changing their minds about what they have learned and everything their community may have been telling them about you as a queer person.

Knowing this, many people choose to be patient with their teammates who are having a hard time adjusting to the fact that you are being open about your sexual identity. While there's no shame in being patient and trying to help people overcome their homophobia or transphobia, there's no reason why you have to take abuse from a person who is supposed to be an ally of yours. You are still a human being and deserve the same respect you had always been given by your teammates, and reminding them of that fact is going to possibly be necessary to ensure that you're not going to be bullied by anyone. If you can do this while there are other teammates nearby to support you when you address homophobia on your team that would be best, just to ensure that the issue does not immediately escalate and that the person you're addressing realizes that the team agrees with your position and that the attacks have to stop.

Remember why you came out and why you play sports at all, if you find that it's just too difficult to be part of a team or that coming out has not given you what you hoped it would from the team and those around the team, you can always find other places to play that will be more welcoming to you. Sports are great, and I do encourage everyone to get involved from as young an age as possible, both for physical health reasons and social reasons, but at the end of the day they are just a fun extra-curricular activity that we all do. It should be fun, and if it's no longer fun after coming out and trying to address the issues being continually brought up by your team, it may be time to find another place to play; there will always be other teams and leagues who will be happy to have you, and your happiness should be the ultimate priority.

I confess this part isn't for everyone; I get that some people aren't interested in being activists and that they would rather just get to work on their athletics without having to worry about anything else that might be happening around them. There's nothing wrong with that, you have to decide what is best for you when you're attempting to be an openly queer athlete, and that may mean that it's best for you to leave the activism and work convincing other people to accept you to other people around you. For those who feel more interested in taking a stand and being involved as more than just an athlete, this section is for you and will talk a bit about how to be an activist without creating too many tense situations with your team and the people surrounding you. Remember, it's still just sports and you are supposed to be there for the sports first and foremost!

Being open about who you are and not backing down when others attempt to make you feel bad for who you are is a great way to start being an agent of change in the athletic world. People are going to make assumptions about you because of the stereotypes we have in the world, and the only real way to deal with stereotypes is to live your life normally and prove that a stereotype is just that, a caricature that doesn't encompass who people really are or what their real skills may be. A lot of the time you're going to want to fight back against the stereotypes and start telling people that they're wrong and what they say is hurtful and not based in reality. That can be helpful and sometimes it is worth saying that what they're saying is wrong, but people don't often like being told straight to their faces that they're wrong, so they can end up being defensive about their beliefs and become less willing to hear what you have to say about why their stereotypes are wrong to begin with. These sorts of people are only ever going to change their mind by seeing the evidence of their own eyes; this means just being proud of yourself and not taking their grief, but not letting them bait you into an argument that will likely solidify their beliefs.

Athletes who come out inevitably spend a lot of time defending who they are to the people around them; teammates, coaches, parents, and if you're high enough up the ladder even the media will start questioning how you can be queer and an athlete at the same time, since they're so often assumed to be totally different and divorced from one another. Take these moments as the opportunities for teaching and learning that they are; the people who are saying these things are often already on your side, but they need more information in order to truly be good allies to you and to support what you're doing by being out while participating in sports. Gently correcting people who make assumptions and explaining how those assumptions are wrong in general or that they don't apply to all people is always going to be helpful, especially if you can find that you can relate it to stereotypes they may have heard about other groups that they know are false. It's also important to make sure that you don't allow yourself to be slandered by anyone, and that they don't have the opportunity to denigrate you or otherwise cause you grief because of your sexual identity.

Depending on how hard you want to push for total acceptance and celebration of queer athletes, you may find that it's worthwhile to try and have your team meet with and partner with queer organizations that also play the same sport as you. Most larger urban areas will have a few queer sports leagues devoted to some of the more popular games in your area, so it can be possible for you to get your team to meet with another team and just share experiences and have the queer league explain some of why they're separate and why it's so important to be able to participate in athletics. Beyond being an opportunity to share stories and have more queer athletes be introduced to your team and showing that the stereotype is not true, it also provides an opportunity for mentoring in terms of the athletic capabilities of your team; they can learn from the queer league's players and try to learn new techniques or practice their fundamentals with a different set of eyes making sure that they are doing it properly.

Attending and participating in pride parades is one of the highlights of everyone's year. The parades are always fun and inclusive of all people, and it is incredibly affirming to be part of a celebration of who we are as queer people and how far we've come in terms of obtaining societal acceptance. People from around the city attend pride parades to show their support for queer acceptance in society, and sometimes just to enjoy the atmosphere and have a good time at the day long events. Pride parades used to be a means of expressing ourselves and our need to be visible and seen in the community so that the rest of society could learn to see that we're no different from they are and deserve equal rights and respect. That's still the main reason that we have pride parades, and in many places around the world it remains true that queer people can be jailed or even executed for being true to themselves.

We're lucky that in the Western world we generally have protections from being hurt or assaulted because of how we identify. There's still much that we do have to accomplish, including protections from discrimination in the workplace and the rest of civil society, but we no longer have to fear for our lives and live in fear that the state will punish us for who we happen to be. More than that, we're struggling to achieve real equality that comes from true understandings of the people instead of just having laws that protect us; it's the difference between tolerance and real acceptance and we're starting to push for that in all areas of society. This has meant pushing the boundaries in some areas that we have yet to be accepted, such as athletics, and is why there remains so much interest whenever there are queer athletes who come out or any support is shown to the queer community from the athletic community.

Attending a pride parade as an athlete and seeing other athletes, both queer and heterosexual, marching in the parade helps create a statement to the rest of society that it's okay to be gay and sporty, and that there's nothing that says you have to be one or the other. Fighting these stereotypes in an incredibly public venue such as a pride parade, which can have thousands of people attending and spectating each year, is not something that's done lightly, but it can be incredibly affirming and demonstrative of how one person or a small group of people can start bringing about societal change. Having people see that there are so many queer athletes who are proud to be seen and identified as having a dual identity of an athlete and a queer person will help cause people to reflect on their assumptions about what it means to be queer and what it means to be an athlete, and by doing so it presents an opportunity to get through to those people and explain to them that the stereotypes they may have grown up with are a caricature that does not always exist in reality.

Coaching is the weak link in the story of greater acceptance of queer athletes in society. Players, owners and the fans seem ready to accept professional athletes who identify as part of the queer spectrum, but there remains a lack of training that's given to coaches to help them prepare for the inevitable and to be able to handle having a queer player of their own. There is currently no material available to help openly gay or closeted coaches determine the best way of coming out to your teams once you're comfortable to do so. Even more importantly, there's absolutely no material available for coaches that have queer athletes on their own team and how to properly adjust their methods in order to be fair to all members of their team. This means that those players who do come out are going to be at a severe disadvantage unless they have a coach that already has training or experience working with queer players, and will only serve to reinforce the notion that athletics is institutionally hostile to queer players. Addressing this situation requires effort on behalf of the national coaching organizations that has yet to be done so far for any sport, including sports that are traditionally seen as more likely to have queer athletes already part of the culture of that sport, such as men's figure skating.

The status of coaches has become static in the last few years as well, there's very little innovation being done in terms of how we deliver lessons and instruction to players, with most of the energy being put forward in the national coaching associations being put towards streamlining services and creating uniform guidelines between the provinces. While there are certainly good reasons for doing so, the least of which being that it ensures quality throughout North America and ensures that players are not disadvantaged because of where they live within

Canada or America, this has meant that there's no change being made to address new and evolving issues in coaching.

One of the main components of coaching in North America has always been an ethical component, ensuring that coaches pass certain guidelines for behaviour governing their interactions with their players and other members of the community, which is especially important when dealing with child athletes. These rules have consistently been put in place to protect both the players and the coaches from any potential problems, and they cover a wide variety of topics to ensure that there is as little potential for mischief as possible between players and coaches. For most coaches, these courses are taken simply because they have to be and it never becomes an issue once they begin coaching their players, but for some coaches it does become an issue. These courses are updated over time to address changes in athletic culture, but there's been nothing so far that would help with the increasing number of queer athletes and queer coaches. This would be the ideal place for any new training regarding queer issues to be placed in the coaching curriculum, and it needs to be addressed with both the provincial and national coaching organizations that govern such policy changes.

Coaches themselves seem to be coming more and more from the ranks of parents that just want to get involved with their children, instead of having people who are actually skilled at the sport and can actively demonstrate the skills and techniques needed to improve the abilities of the players on the team. There's nothing wrong with this, and there's actually a great deal of good that can be done by having parents be more active in the lives of their players, but it also presents a series of concerns that players may not be treated fairly because of any connections they may have to the coach. It's not something that parents obviously intend to do, but there is always that lingering suspicion that needs to be addressed about whether parents are getting involved for everyone on the team or to ensure that their own child gets good playing time. The converse of this is that more professional coaches with no connection to the team may not be willing to make the long term commitments needed to bring teams who wish to be competitive up to the level they want to be at. For teams that are more recreational or who aren't as concerned with advancing to an elite level, but it remains something to be considered if the players are going to stay together and they're continually adjusting to new coaches and coaching styles each year.

Having been a coach in both situations and a player in both situations with parents and professionals as coaches, I find that it's easier to be a coach when you don't know the players and can't base your understanding of the players on anything you might already know about their personalities. It makes things a bit more difficult in the beginning of your tenure as coach when you're trying to sort out personalities and skill levels for your players, but it's important to go into the process without any preconceptions of what any of the players are capable of doing or what you can do to motivate them to succeed. Learning all of this through firsthand experiences and through interactions with the players is a key part of how we forge strong connections with those players and have them trust you when their trust is needed. This is particularly true for queer coaches who are considering coming out to their teams and need to ensure that there will be a community environment that is trusting and open to communicating about concerns and personal issues that might otherwise derail the ability for a coach and team to communicate with one another. Even for coaches who aren't contemplating coming out or who have already come out to their team, forging and maintaining these connections is of vital importance to maintaining your ability to get through to the players and have them feel interested in learning from you and respecting the way you choose to lead the team.

Coaches themselves are also not committing to their teams as much as they otherwise should and that the players are coming to expect regular changes in coaches when they participate in team sports. Whether it's because a parent coach leaves because their child is no longer participating or the more professional coach is unable to commit for another year, players have started taking it as a given that their coach won't be returning the following year. This has meant that in many sports there's now a lack of trained coaches available who are willing to take on teams, and players are being turned away from lack of anyone to help run the team and provide the certification needed to be acceptable to the organizing authorities for that sport. This tends to hamper the ability for players to develop their skills in a consistent manner and instead leads to a significant amount of wasted time trying to bring the coaches and players in sync with one another.

For teams interested in competing at higher levels, this is unacceptable and can stagnate the team's progress while their competitors continue to improve and gain more experience together that can be useful at important competitions. It often takes a significant amount of time to get comfortable coaching a new team, and that has to do with both how you teach them and their willingness to listen to you beyond just understanding what your qualifications are to be there as their coach; having to continually go through that partnership process and learning process with a team means that less time is spent working on skills and providing teams with games they can use to work together and effectively makes the team less able to prepare for competitions. Younger teams especially need the time to prepare for competition and feel certain that there's compatibility between themselves and the coaching staff.

As a first year curling coach with a brand new team, I found it was very difficult for my team to get motivated to prepare for an upcoming bonspiel that they were registered to play in. Not because they weren't excited to be in a competitive situation and to prepare for their end of season championships; they were quite excited about that, but because I was a new coach to them and they were a new team that was just learning to mesh with each other, that comfort level wasn't there and there were persistent concerns of being unprepared that I wasn't able to effectively deal with. Those concerns grew in scope as the bonspiel approached, and while they accepted that I was their coach, they were still nervous about how they would perform and honestly how I would perform as their coach, both during the games when I would be unable to help them directly and then between games when I would be responsible for talking over how the game went and preparing them mentally and physically for the next game a few hours later.

As it turns out, things went relatively well, though I feel that I wasn't able to adequately get my players to take me seriously because of how new I was to being their coach. This was compounded a bit by the fact that their former coach was at the same bonspiel with his new team, and they were still able to talk with him and get his perspective on a number of things that I wanted to bring up without interference from another source. As the season continued on and I was able to get more involved with the team and their practices and games, they really started to trust what I was saying and doing, and they did start improving significantly more than they were at the beginning of the year when they weren't as attuned to my way of coaching and how I wanted to demonstrate skills to them. This trust became important once we were at the end of year championships and they were having to play multiple games in a single day; they were eager to hear what I had to say in regards to how they played the previous game, what went wrong, what went right and how to prepare for the next game, including their nutritional needs and an opportunity to relax and relieve stress before heading back out on the ice. None of that would have been possible if I hadn't been able to create a stronger connection with them, which also meant that the following year produced even better results for the team once I was back and able to get back into coaching them.

Working as a coach inevitably means that you will have to build a working or tolerable relationship with your players parents or significant others, most of whom are going to be in regular attendance at your games and practices and who are all likely to have their own views on what should be done in order to make the team or more likely their specific player that they know improve and get more playing time. This can be one of the most difficult parts of coaching to ensure that all players receive a fair amount of playing time and that everyone has a chance to develop at their own pace, while also ensuring that the team is able to reach is competitive goals. How you address that balance is dependent on the kind of team you're coaching and even the ages of the players. Obviously when the players are younger and just starting in the sport it is far more important to ensure everyone gets an equitable amount of playing time and that everyone gets to play every position and find what works best for them. On the other hand, older players may be more willing to accept differing levels of playing time, particularly if they are playing in a position that requires less playing time to be effective.

Near the end of my baseball career, I started seeing significantly less playing time and found that I was willing to accept that as a part of my athletic life. I was on a competitive team and was still playing well, but I had begun to specialize as a member of the pitching staff and thus was not needed to play every single inning. I found that there were many games where I didn't play at all, just because of the numbers we had and the need to ensure everyone was well-rested as part of the league rules regarding how much a person can pitch in a single week. So my playing time did fall by a significant amount compared to when I was younger, but because I had begun to specialize it wasn't meant as a means of stating that I was harming the team's chances for success. By contrast, in my curling life I play significantly less than I did earlier in my curling career, and that's because everyone does everyone else's job very effectively, and the number of people on our team is enough that I'm not needed to play each day.

The balance between equitable playing time and the needs of the team to succeed change somewhat when working with a high performance or other competitive team. Time should always be spent developing the skills of all players on the team, but there also begins to be an understanding that certain people are more successful in high stress situations such as important games or critical moments within games, and players on these higher performance teams will be more likely to understand that the team's needs will sometimes outweigh their own personal needs or wishes. Should any kind of situation arise where substitutions are needed, ensure that the parents and the players themselves know that it's not anything personal about the player and is not meant to signal that you don't have faith in that player, it's a professional decision that you're doing to help everyone on the team succeed. This can be hard to do, especially when a player hasn't done anything they believe to be wrong or feel that they are being played less than they should be compared to some of their peers. Addressing these perceived biases and the suggestion that you are playing favourites is something that has to be dealt with immediately, both for the sake of your professional reputation and for the players to trust the decisions that you are making.

Early in my own baseball career, I was always on the bubble to make the competitive team; every other year I would be cut and sent down to the house league team, and in the years that I was not cut I often did not see very much playing time because of how my skills compared to the rest of my team. While it could be argued that my reduced playing time made it more difficult to catch up to my teammates, I did get equal skill development time during practices, it was just that during game situations I was not as skilled as my peers and wasn't able to contribute as effectively to the success of the team. One year at provincials, I had been playing in the outfield, which was where you stuck the weaker members of the team at the time, and the next inning I was told I would be substituted for another member of the team. We were getting late in the game and it was still close, and the coaches knew that I wasn't the best batter or fielder at the time. By substituting me they gave the team an opportunity to have a better batter take my place, and someone who was roughly at the same calibre in terms of fielding. As it turned out, the substitution didn't work as expected and we did end up losing that game, and at the time it felt like I was being taken off because I wasn't one of the coach's favourite players. In hindsight, I realize that my skills were not where they needed to be for a provincial championship and that I probably did contribute as much as I could at that point in my playing career. The whole situation could have been dealt with better by the coaches if they had been able or willing to explain why they had taken me out, beyond telling me that it was time to come off and be substituted in for someone else.

Parents and other spectators are unlikely to understand those kinds of balancing acts that you have to do in the course of being a coach for their charges, they're likely just to see that you aren't treating everyone equally or that you're squandering an opportunity to win in order to make sure everyone gets a chance without regard for how doing so may impact the team. More often than not, you're not going to have the time to explain to each aggrieved person why the person they care about is playing too much or too little, and even more than that you won't have the time to explain each piece of strategy or choice of tactics you make during the course of a game or season. The only real thing you can do is try to be honest with people with the most pressing or legitimate concerns, and if possible try to deal with more than one concern at a time if they are related or similar to each other. If parents or other adults continue to question you or otherwise undermine your authority with the players, it may become suitable to invite them to join you and have them assist you, that way they can have more input and see how coaching is done from your own perspective and start to understand the reason why you do what you do, and how they could potentially improve or not improve on your decisions.

In terms of coming out to the parents or significant others on the team you're coaching, doing so earlier in the season is the best opportunity to do so. It shows the parents that you have nothing to hide and that you're only intentions are to provide skills and leadership to your charges, and sadly also gives the parents time to remove their child if their beliefs will not allow them to have you work with their child. Like many other groups or individuals you will come out to over the course of your life, the people connected to your players will also likely have questions for you about you being queer and also heavily involved in sports. Some will even make stereotyped assumptions about your purpose in the locker room or other places where there is the potential for problematic situations arising between you and the players. These kinds of comments have to be taken in stride and plans have to be made to show that you don't believe this is a concern for those parents. For sports that do require full changing before and after games, this might mean something as simple as having a separate office or locker room for yourself and the rest of the adult coaching staff, or it may mean that you have to wait to change out of your gear until after everyone has left or in the privacy of your own home. Having these plans and being comfortable sharing with the parents of your players how you're going to ensure that there are no crossed boundaries will go far in relaxing the parents and having them trust you, as will coming out voluntarily instead of being forced out by other people who may have an agenda against you.

If you already have experience being a coach or serving in another position that put you in a position of authority over youth or other potential players you might coach, having people from that workplace or situation provide character references for you can be an additional means of showing to concerned parents and guardians that you are able to be trusted by them. These references can come from almost anywhere, including the staff of the organization or association you're coaching with, any past organizations you worked for, or if you teach as your profession or do something in your professional life that involves working with and caring for others, references from those locations can also serve to put the minds of others at ease that you can be trusted and will respect all boundaries that need to be respected between a player and coach. That isn't to say that you need to provide a full resume and set of references for each and every person that has a complaint or concern about your ability to maintain professional distance between you and those around you, but it can serve as a means of placating those who have not worked with you before.

New coaches don't have that same luxury to be able to call upon past years of serving in the organization and the trust that comes from being a familiar face among the parents who have been raising their children in the sport or for adults who have been playing in the league for an extended period of time. For these people, they are less likely to accept you at face value because you are new and don't have a past reputation to fall back upon that these people will immediately recognize, and any external references you have will not be something they can corroborate with their own past experiences with you or around you in the league. Being open to hearing these people's concerns and explaining how you will address them can help show them your intentions towards the players. As with many other situations involving skeptical outsiders, the best thing to do is to invite them to see your practice and observe for themselves how you act around the players and other parents on the team. This can sometimes be disruptive but it does show that you're willing to be accommodating, and unfortunately there are still many people who believe in stereotypes about queer people who will need to be convinced by their own experiences that you can be trusted and are capable of both providing the skills the players need and also to be a proper role model for the players. Alternatively, and this may appeal to new coaches in particular, working with other coaches that do have that kind of reputation and track record can serve as a means of building that reputation for yourself. This might be a situation where you would serve as the assistant coach to a more familiar or entrenched coach, and build from there towards coaching your own team once the numbers allow for it and there's greater comfort in your abilities to coach a team and work without other coaches ensuring you're demonstrating the skills properly.

However you choose to address the myriad concerns that parents and other fans are likely to bring to your attention as the coach, it is important to ensure that you treat all parents fairly and that you also do not take out any feelings you may have from being questioned out on the players themselves. The players have to continually be the main focus of your attention, and diverting yourself away from the players to address the concerns of parents or others is a distraction that your players don't deserve. Further to that, it goes without saying that you can't punish the player for something their parent or friend might say or imply about your abilities or anything else that may be brought up by those people; they're doing what they think they have to in order to protect their friend or child, and that sometimes means they do things that are not acceptable or wise. It's hard to say and harder to do while it's happening, but ignoring it and moving on as quickly as possible once you have time to address their concerns is the best thing to do and will reduce the time spent away from your actual coaching priorities.

Trust is an integral part of being an effective coach. Without the ability for your players to trust you, it will be impossible for them to really take to heart the messages that you are giving them and attempting to instil into them, whether they're interpersonal or athletic in nature. Creating this trust with your new players is a cycle that can be difficult to start and harder still to maintain in the face of adversity and confusion from your charges. For your players, it becomes difficult for them to trust you unless you give them reasons to start trusting you, and the converse of that is that it is difficult to give the players a reason to trust you when you have only just met them and don't trust how they will react around you. Working your way into trusting each other with small acts that show you're genuine and mean the best for their personal and professional growth will build that relationship over time. This relationship and trust is important if you are planning to come out to your players, particularly when working with younger players who you hold a position of authority over.

How you create those safe spaces is entirely up to you, different coaches and coaching styles will have different ideas for how you should tell your players that you're available to be an adult they can talk to if they're having problems, and there's no right or wrong way to show that you're on their side and want to help them get through whatever is bothering them. Many coaches find that they don't even have to specifically state that they can be seen as an adult to come talk to when it's needed, the players themselves will just naturally do so if you're able to create a good relationship with them and earn a reputation for being fair minded and willing to hear their side of the issue without prejudice or dismissing them out of hand. The important thing is how you follow through on those words and policies and ensure that you're actually able to contribute the help that you say you're able to do. This will mean hearing things that you might not be prepared to hear, and knowing how you have to address the potential concerns that come up as part of what the player says to you. If you're working with youth, be aware of what the laws require you to do in your jurisdiction; many states and provinces have laws requiring adults in a position of authority to alert authorities when they are told about abuse or other potential problems that require the intervention of professional services. Knowing how to address those situations without compromising the trust the player has put in you is difficult, but the welfare of the player is the most important thing and you will have to follow whatever policies are put in place by your team or organization, which will be in accordance with local law.

Coming out to youth is an incredibly precarious position that has to be done and is not something that should be done right away with the team. Depending on the age of the players, their level of maturity and the family backgrounds they come from, it may be difficult to come out at all and that can present a barrier to you as you try and forge genuine connections with your players. From the perspective of gaining their trust and having them work with you in a way that is beneficial to both the players and yourself, it is probably best to come out to your players eventually. What should be done first is to talk to the parents about the situation and come out to them first; they may have their own reservations about you telling their sons or daughters about that part of your personal life and believe that it isn't something that the players need to know in order to listen to you. If that becomes the case then it's important to take that information and follow through with it instead of telling the players behind the backs of the parents; that too is a loss of trust that will damage the team in the end.

Assuming that the parents aren't concerned about you coming out to their children and the players remain on the team, the actual art of coming out to a player or team is a bit more difficult than it would be when you are the player or coming out to someone else. As a coach, your main duty is to the players themselves, and as a volunteer you're meant to be working with the youth on their skills, A coming out scenario that focuses all of the attention on you and your own personal issues and need to be out detracts from that for the players and makes it feel that you're the important part of the equation, instead of the players. That cannot happen when you're a coach, that's a fundamental issue that must always be upheld is that you are there for them, they aren't there for you. With that being said, there are always ways of coming out without having to make a scene or take a specific moment to be out and tell your players. More useful would be the concept where you drop hints about your sexual orientation or gender identity and allow your players to draw their own conclusions; it's very likely that if you have an established rapport with your players they will ask you on their own when they feel comfortable to do so, particularly if they are younger and more willing to bring up questions like that.

When that question does come up, whether it's just one player or all the players, it can generally be assumed that the rest of the team is at least somewhat curious and is probably concerned about it to the point where it may be distracting the players from the game and also from taking you as seriously as they should because of the potential for stereotyping. There's also the possibility that your players will be confused about why you held something like that away from them, and in that case it would be a fair time to bring it up and tell your team, since at that point they will be ready to hear it and it should not result in any repercussions. The key is to gauge your players and determine how they're reacting to the news you're giving them; they may have questions or reactions that are not as positive as your coworkers or peers would be, and that's understandable. Work with your players to explain your rationale behind why you didn't tell them and remind them that it's not important to why you're in their lives, it's just a part of yourself that is different from what they may have been expecting from you.

Being a queer coach means more than just ensuring that your personal life is protected and understood by the players and parents of players that you are entrusted with, it also means that you have to actually get out there and help develop the skills of the players that you're working with. This is the fun part of coaching, and also the part that is going to tire you out the most, both physically and mentally as you try and find new ways to demonstrate the skills and keep the players interested. It helps that your players are going to want to listen to what you have to say because you have the experience they need to become better players.

How you teach these skills and interact with your players is of utmost importance, as you will hold a position of authority over them even if you are coaching players in your age range and who are not children. There needs to be an understanding that your players are very likely to understand that you hold some level of power over their ability to play or learn how to improve their skills, and while as a coach it would be unethical to actively try and punish players for how they react to certain situations, it has to be something that is considered when talking to your players, particularly once the topic of discussion becomes your personal life and you consider coming out to your players. Many will be concerned to speak freely for fear that doing so may hamper their ability to get equal playing time if they feel that their answer will not be what you are expecting.

Creating a plan for each practice and game, or any other interaction you're going to have with your players can help ensure that you remain professional with the players and that there are no concerns about any boundaries being crossed between you. More than that, the players have to be aware of what the limits are going to be, especially once you come out to them and those concerns become crystallized in their minds as something that needs to be considered when you and them interact with each other.

Like anything else though, a balance needs to be struck between remaining distant with your players and showing that you're willing to engage with them. Many activities that would be considered inappropriate or potentially awkward outside of sports are completely acceptable on the field, but then would also be considered possibly inappropriate for you to do as an out queer coach. The baseball teams I played on generally had a policy of patting a person's behind when they did a good job or made a good play; this sometimes extended to the coaches themselves, though this was more likely to be because we were dawdling and needed something to get us to move a bit faster, and it became more of a swat than anything else. For heterosexual players and coaches, the gesture looks remarkable boring and tame; it's two players or a player and coach encouraging one another and reminding each other to play hard and relax while doing so. For a queer coach it becomes more open to interpretation as to whether that same action was meant to be encouraging or whether it has other connotations or meanings. This is something you'll have to decide for yourself when you're coaching and determine what you think those boundaries for appropriate behaviour should be among your teammates.

The players themselves are very likely to set the tone for what kind of activities they'll find appropriate, and from there you can just emulate them or find actions that are similar in scope to what they are doing and do those if you prefer.

Your judgment should be relatively good at determining what those limits of professional and personal behaviour should be, but let the players know that you're always open to hearing from them if they feel that something doesn't feel right for them. They may be fine with their teammates acting a certain way, but because you have a position of authority over them and are likely to have a significant age gap between you and them, and that may make something you do feel appropriate to them. First, don't panic. These things happen at times and it's not that you had a malicious intent behind what you did, so you'll need to apologize and explain why you did what you did. Let your player explain why they felt uncomfortable with what you did, and let them get what they need to say off their chest before apologizing and giving your explanation. Once that occurs, you should ask and ensure that no other players are feeling uncomfortable as well, and have the player or players themselves brainstorm things that you could do instead to show your support and encouragement to the players that would not be as intrusive or feel as awkward to them as the action that you did.

The hardest part about maintaining professionalism around your players is going to be when they are complaining to you about play time or other aspects of the sport itself that they feel you are not doing to the best of your ability or that you are otherwise not ensuring that everyone is able to benefit from your coaching equally.

Dismissing their concerns out of hand is not an option, and will only serve to reinforce what they believe about you and make your job more difficult once you are trying to coach them again. Trying to explain your actions can also be problematic when attempting to explain differences in play time with younger players who may just want to know why everyone doesn't just play the same as everyone else. Finding the means to communicate with your players is going to be most difficult at this point, but it's a skill that you need to develop and the best course of action is to consider their needs and points first and foremost, and then decide how to react and explain yourself in a way that won't exacerbate the problems that they have brought to your attention.

In many ways, working with and communicating with parents and other guardians of your players will be easier than working with your players themselves. With the parents and other fans who you will be interacting with, they will be in the same age cohort as yourself and you will have that equal level of respect for one another that comes with being in the same age group. This often will make it easier to talk about potentially difficult issues because you'll already be aware of the other person's likely level of maturity and willingness to understand your point of view. Those fans also have the benefit of being at least partially removed from the situation that is occurring on the field and thus are less likely to react emotionally to what is happening or your responses to those events.

Your players, on the other hand, are not going to be as lucky or as far removed from the situation. They're unfortunately the ones who have to accept the decisions that you make and are not always able to understand why you are making those decisions. Younger players in particular are not going to be emotionally mature enough to discuss things with you in the same manner you would talk to their parents or their guardians, and this means that you must find a different way to approach topics with the players that ensures they understand what is going on and why things are done they way they are being done without becoming condescending or talking over their heads. This will often depend on what exactly is being discussed and the circumstances in which it became an issue between you and the player or players.

When addressing concerns related to the sport itself and how the team will be run, it makes the most sense just to be straightforward and direct in what you are going to do. This works for both junior and adult players, and having those clear expectations be set from the beginning of the season will help curtail any problems that may occur later in the year. In general, players will be coming into the team with at least some kind of expectation and understanding of what acceptable behaviour would be, and they won't have to be told too much about what they are expected to do from you, but having those reminders done at the beginning of the year will make the rest of the season go forward more smoothly.

With regards to dealing with coaching issues and the players themselves, the most common and often the most difficult part of coaching will be defusing conflicts between players on your team. Addressing player concerns about playing time or the way in which skills are being developed in practices are easier to deal with and can be explained by talking about the methodology you learned in your coaching courses that explain why you're doing things in a certain step by step formula. Players will often accept those as facts, and the building of those foundational skills towards more specialized skills will make sense to the players once they get to the point where they are actually learning those higher level sports skills and realising that it would not have been possible to accomplish those skills without the basic skills that were taught earlier in the year or in past years by previous coaches. This is also true of playing time conflicts, where it becomes even easier to notice that there are only so many positions on the court and that there are often more players on the team than there are positions, so at some point someone is going to have to take a break and not play, at least in the short term.

On the other hand, working out differences between players who are fighting with each other can be quite difficult, particularly when one or both of the players involved feels that they have done nothing wrong and when they are younger players who are involved in the fight. Finding ways of ensuring that both sides are able to save face should be the paramount goal of the conflict resolution strategies you use, and the secondary goal should be to determine how that and similar situations are not brought up again on the team. It's been my own experience that the best way of ensuring that the fights are dealt with is to be blunt with the players in question and not back down from whatever your decision happens to be; this is particularly true when the issue is a matter is personal in nature and does not have to do with the sport or the team itself, and is confined to how those two players see each other and their lack of respect for one another.

When I was a player on my midget baseball team, a teammate and I had a fight at the beginning of one of our seasons, and it became problematic enough that it affected our ability to play and be part of the same team, and actually devolved at one point into a shouting match between us while we were both trying to play our respective positions at that point in time. As it was the first game in a double-header for us, at the end of the game the coach told us both to leave and work out our issues with each other, and not to return to the bench until we were satisfied that we could work with each other and respect one another enough to at least get through the next game without fighting or creating a dramatic scene that would take away from the team's ability to concentrate on the game. I remember at the time I was livid about being banished because of how my teammate had been treating me and how he was focusing on criticizing me instead of trying to support me. Being isolated from the rest of the team gave us both an opportunity to be completely candid with one another and while we still disliked each other for the rest of the time we played with each other, we both realized that we weren't helping our team by being forcibly removed from the active roster, and decided that the best thing to do was to try and ignore one another until we had an opportunity to settle down and face our issues with a bit less emotion behind our actions.

Interpersonal problems are not the only place as a coach that you will have to deal with your players in an age appropriate way. For queer coaches, how we come out to our teams is of vital importance, and is something that has to be done delicately in order to ensure that everyone remains respectful and that there are no concerns or hard feelings among any of the people present when you come out to them. Older players are more likely to react with what they believe are the stereotypes about queer people, and these are concerns that you will have to address. Teenage players are especially more likely to think about potential stereotypes because of the peer pressure they are likely to be feeling to conform to the image of an athlete or jock, which has often meant a certain degree of heteronormativity and flaunting of their male and heterosexual sexuality. Coming out to them and maintaining a position of authority over these kinds of jock players will present a conflict for them and puts into question some of their previously held beliefs about queer people. This conflict can sometimes mean they will rebel in order to try and assert their dominance as jocks and as heterosexuals who believe that queer people are out of place in the athletic world. Younger players are more likely to react with confusion, as they may not be aware of divergent sexualities and sexual orientations, so by coming out you may be creating a situation where you are introducing orientations that they were not aware of or did not know were to be found in human society, against the wishes of their parents.

Addressing how teens react to your coming out will be based mainly on how they choose to see you and whether they see your minority orientation as a threat to their own sexuality as male or female athletes who are presumably heterosexual and participate in sports in order to help affirm that sexuality. Speaking with your players about how nothing is really changing and honestly answering any questions they may have will help with your players' attitudes towards you now that they will be aware of your sexual orientation or gender identity. However, this is not meant to say that you should create an open invitation for your players to ask you anything about your personal life and the contents of your life away from sports;

you have the right to keep some aspects of yourself private and away from the players' knowledge, particularly when it is not relevant to your ability to coach them or to your being a queer coach. Teenaged players may also feel that this gives them an opportunity to try and rebel against some of the things you have been doing as part of your coaching duties; this is just an attempt to challenge your authority and should not be permitted to continue, as doing so will hurt your ability to maintain a good coaching relationship with the team. Reminding your players that you still have a lot to teach them about the sport itself is also helpful in trying to retain control of the situation and prevent your players from disrespecting you as a response to your coming out. In general the best decision to take with regards to teenage players is to be honest but also to ensure they know when they have pushed too far.

Younger players will require a bit more tact than to simply tell them that you are queer and that you are going to be staying on as their coach. With younger players who may not know exactly what it means to be a member of the queer community or even what the definitions of some of the identities we have for ourselves, it can often be overwhelming to learn that your coach or another person in authority lives their lives in a way that is different from what they have known and likely grown up with. The safest thing to do is to tell the parents that you are planning on coming out to your team first, and let them take the lead on how they think you should best come out to the players. This may mean that you simply tell the players that you are queer and then allow the parents to define that term how they choose to do so as a private family matter, or it may mean that the parents will want to be present for that particular point in the practice or after a game so that they can ensure you do not say things that will lead to too many questions that the parents are not ready to answer from their children. Getting too detailed in what it means to be queer is going to be too much for younger players to understand and deal with, and will likely just lead to situations where they feel uncomfortable playing on the team because of tension that may exist either between you and the player or between you and their parents. A significant amount of preparation will have to be done in concert with the parents before coming out to younger players, and it may be decided by the families of those players that it is not something you should do at all. If that does become the case where the parents have reservations about you coming out to the team, their decision should be respected, as it is not your right to interfere with how those parents raise their children, no matter how you may disagree or how it may affect you personally by having to force yourself into the closet. Staying in the closet often ends up being easier for coaches of younger players as well, as they are not especially interested in your personal life and are unlikely to be asking about what you do outside of coaching them, so there won't be as likely a need to lie or fabricate stories about who you spend your time with and how you spend your time with them. Reminding yourself that you are there in order to teach skills will be the most important part of maintaining age appropriate conversations with your younger players, and in particular when dealing with issues of sexuality and your potential coming out to the team.

Beyond the players, the fans and the parents who you will have to defend yourself to and constantly be aware of when you make decisions for the team, the other people you have to be in constant communication with and have a strong relationship with are the other members of the coaching staff. Whether you're coaching a recreational curling team or an elite baseball team headed for provincials, there's a lot more to it than just the one coach who's in charge of the team. You have assistant coaches, managers, people serving as a liaison with your association, someone working with the league to ensure the team remains under the proper guidelines, and even team parents who help provide transportation and food for the players between games and to and from their games and practices. All these people have to be working in sync with each other, and that means having good communication with them and being able to trust one another. These are also people with whom you have to be willing to tell about your sexual orientation or gender identity, and you have to be able to trust them that they won't try to make your life difficult by doing so, which is a consideration that you have to think about before taking on the responsibility of coming out to anyone else related or associated with the team.

Some of these people will be people you probably already know; you may have people who are already going to be part of your staff team that you know from your own experiences and who already know that you identify as part of the queer community. Others will be people who you haven't met before, and who may be people you haven't even seen in the association before and who are only recently deciding to step up and volunteer to help out with their child or friend's team. The kind of community and relationship you create with these people will be determined by your initial meetings with the group and how you explain what each person's role is likely to be with the team. Working with these newer volunteers is quite satisfying, but can sometimes be exhausting as they are very well-meaning, but ultimately do not always know what it is they have to do in order to complete the goals and responsibilities of their job. These kinds of parents will be looking to you for support and guidance on how to ensure they do their jobs for the team effectively and without becoming overly taxed themselves. Parents that have been doing volunteer work for a number of years will be a different kind of challenge, as they will be looking to see how well you are able to mesh with the rest of the adult staff and see if you do things that are very different from what they are used to from other coaches and teams.

Working within the group requires effective communication, and in general that shouldn't be too much of a problem; everyone is there to benefit the players of the team, and as volunteers there aren't usually too many strong egos involved to create power dynamics that are not in the best interests of the team. Where this can go astray is with your coming out, for many of the same reasons that it would provide problems with the rest of the parents on the team. Where there may be a difference for these involved parents and those who are just fans who watch their players is that they are more involved and will be able to see you on a more frequent basis interacting with the players and the rest of the people associated with the league, and thus would be in a better position to judge how you act and whether any potential concerns could arise between you and the players.

Find a way to work with these active volunteers and have them explain any concerns they may have when you initially come out to them, and explain that you're informing them first to ensure that there won't be any potential problems between you and anyone else associated with the team. In this case, your proactive stance will be interpreted as being helpful and trying to ensure that the team operates smoothly and doesn't require any additional concerns to occur at a more important date, such as when the team is trying to focus on important games or their playoff season. To that end, coming out to your support staff and volunteers should be done early in the year and after a practice or some other moment when the staff will be together and separated from the players and their families, so that any concerns that may erupt between the staff of the team can remain separate from the rest of the players and families and can be addressed before they become a problem for everyone else.

Doing this as a stand alone meeting between the staff members on the team is the best solution, as this will leave everyone ample opportunity to discuss any issues they may have and will also mean that the people involved in the meeting will not be distracted by having to watch over the players or equipment. This will also ensure that the initial meeting and concerns remain private and are not heard by anyone else who may not be ready to hear about your coming out or who may not need to know about it right away. Make clear that you have no intention of standing down and resigning as the coach of the team, but that you want to hear from everyone who you will be working with what their concerns are and what potential solutions they may have that can help rectify the situation or at least ameliorate the problem in such a way that everyone is able to perform their duties for the team without any noticeable changes that can be picked up on by those who are not at the meeting. By committing yourself to open communication between yourself and the rest of the staff, you will provide an opportunity for everyone to be assured that you will be taking their concerns into consideration, and then it becomes important to follow through on what is told to you and create an action plan for yourself and the rest of the staff that can be followed to ensure that these concerns about your sexuality are addressed, along with any concerns you may have with the rest of the adults helping you and how they may treat you as a result of coming out. Most teams and situations will find that it's not necessary to create a written contract that details everyone's new roles as a result of coming out, since most people are usually willing to accommodate changes and diversity, or at least tolerate it for the sake of the team and the players' ability to perform as well as they should. If it becomes necessary, a written contract can always be written by the parties involved in the discussion and who have concerns, and future meetings throughout the year can always be scheduled between you and the rest of the staff to ensure that everyone feels as though they are being heard and that the agreements put into place are being followed appropriately.

I did my first coaching certification in 2010. I'm looking at recertifying and upgrading my certification right now, and while the name of the specific coaching level I would be receiving has changed, what has not changed is the way that we teach people to become coaches and the material that is covered as part of the certification process. This is a bit of a shame, because many of the issues that used to be brought up in coaching ethics classes are still relevant, there are a number of issues that are being ignored and considered not worth any time to discuss with coaches who may be new to the system, or even coaches who have been working with athletes for a number of years or decades. We teach coaches how to be ethical in the context of proper relationships with their players and how to ensure that players are being honest with themselves and the league. We teach coaches about the need for proper nutrition and health and wellness training for higher performance teams. We even teach a little bit about interpersonal dynamics and conflict resolution, as well as the need to follow the law and ensure everything done by the team is above board and not in violation of any laws or regulations of the league your team participates in.

What isn't covered in any section of the course, either theoretical or practical, is how to address queer issues that are quickly becoming a major part of the conversation in North American athletic circles. More and more athletes are coming out, and they're doing so at all levels of athletics, including some that are now professional athletes. Coaching hasn't changed to address this critical concern of how to coach a queer player and ensure that they are still respected and treated the same way as everyone else on the team, the same way that gender issues are still not readily discussed in coaching courses for co-ed or potentially mixed gender sports like curling or swimming. In general, the coaching certification process assumes everyone who wears the team's uniform are absolutely similar to each other in all ways, or if they are different those differences are considered unimportant and not worth discussing in any context other than to note that those differences exist on some level that is not related to athletics or coaching at all. This is a ridiculous viewpoint and flies in the face of the idea of a multicultural and diverse society that we happen to live in, and doesn't do anything to prepare coaches for working with people who are not exactly like themselves. Since we don't live in a society of clones, coaches should be given training on how to address issues of diversity that may come up during the course of an athletic season.

This generally has meant a discussion of different ethnic, cultural and religious differences that could contribute to players being absent on certain days or being unable to participate in certain activities because of their beliefs. There are also small sections in the nutrition and wellness section of the courses that cover nutrition for people whose beliefs will not allow them to eat certain kinds of foods, but this too is placed entirely within the context of the sport and maximizing the player's potential to be a good athlete. These discussions ignore the context in which people participate in sports, which is that it is a group activity and meant to be a social activity done with other people and which has the possibility for conflict to occur because of those differences that we are not learning about how to mitigate as coaches.

It is from these interpersonal connections and conflicts that our coaching education courses need to be vastly improved, and that includes having a section devoted to the needs of queer players and coaches, all of whom are routinely ignored as part of the training process and are assumed to not exist at all. In particular, something that would be of use to both queer and heterosexual coaches is information on how to react and what to do if and when a player comes out to them and needs support from the team. When I was playing, I was always concerned about how my coaches would react if I were to come out, and as a result I never actually told any of my coaches that I was gay, and instead hid it so that only players in my own age group and who I trusted would know. I had no reason to assume that the coaching staff would be instinctively supportive of me because I was stuck believing my own stereotypes about the people involved in athletics, and thus was not able to get my coaches to support me and make the transition out of the closet easier for me.

What could be done is to create scenarios where people come out to each other as part of the coaching course, and there could be a discussion between the facilitators and those who were in attendance at the course as to how those players could be supported. This might mean having current queer athletes or coaches come in to the course and provide their own input with how would be best to address the issues of a queer player, or it might mean the creation of completely new curricula created in consultation with queer advocacy groups across the country who would be better able to canvass the needs of queer athletes and coaches than the national coaching organization would be able to do.

Should new curricula be created to address queer issues, coming out and how to address it as both a player and a coach would need to be a fundamental part of the program, but also how to address the issues surrounding fair use of the locker room or change room for those sports that require changing before and after competition. This is of particular concern to members of the transgender community, who are often unsure of which locker room they would be accepted in when preparing for conversation, comparable to how there are often concerns in the transgender community about which washroom to use and how their personal gender identification is not always accepted by the state or society as a whole. Discussions around transgender issues also need to be resolved around which gendered leagues they would be able to participate in, and whether it would be the birth gender or the self-identity that is considered more important for determining which league they would play in. This conversation would also be complicated by the individual situation of each transgender athlete, who may be in varying stages of transitioning from their birth gender to their identified gender and which can create differences in their ability to participate in gendered sports because of the hormonal differences that would lead to biological differences. The preferable solution here would be to allow participants to participate in the gendered league most aligned with the person's gender identity, and that birth biology is an insufficient reason to bar people from participating in the league they would feel most comfortable in. This too is something that would have to be discussed at the national level in order to ensure that there was a uniform decision that all groups would accept instead of leaving it up to each local sports association to decide for themselves.

Something that hasn't come up often is the idea of athletes who have queer parents, as opposed to being queer themselves. Particularly now that marriage equality is a fact of life in Canada and is becoming increasingly accepted in the United States, the number of children being raised with same sex parents is increasing, and is something that coaches should be trained to understand as an acceptable family structure that occurs in society. These families have their own kinds of struggles and it should remain important that the coaching staff of a team learn how to be sensitive to those differences so as to not unintentionally say something that could be perceived as damaging or rude to a child of a same sex family. This would likely look at ensuring that communications requesting help from parents is gender neutral and does not make assumptions about the composition of each family, which should be considered good practice even if it were confirmed that there were no same sex families on the team, as that would also prevent discrimination from occurring against single parents or players being raised by people who are not their immediate family.

Athletics today has changed an awful lot from when I first started getting involved in my beginner leagues and lessons two decades ago. In the mid 1990s queer sexuality was still largely put out of the public eye, or when it was mentioned it was only to reinforce the stereotypes that already existed in the public mind. The idea of queer athletes was almost considered beyond the realm of possibility, even though many former athletes had come out publicly by then; those people were met with absolute shock that they hadn't been completely heterosexual and cisgendered. A lot of that had to do with the fact that in the past, there just weren't many people who were out of the closet at all. You heard about there being a gay person here and there, but it wasn't the kind of cohesive community that exists now, where people could see that we were a significant minority group that made up a large segment of the population. We also didn't know back then why people were gay, and there was a lot of stigma attached because of old stereotypes that no longer exist in most of today's society.

The situation now is quite different and much more sympathetic and supportive of queer athletes. We have college athletes coming out of the closet to their teams while still active players and not being punished for it at all, either directly because of fears and homophobia or indirectly by reducing their playing time or ability to succeed at their chosen sport. Instead, these athletes are being celebrated for their honesty to their teammates and their talent on the field. We are even beyond the point now where we praise gay athletes for their courage in coming out; it's becoming a common enough occurrence and society has become so comfortable with the idea of openly queer people that coming out itself is no longer being considered a heroic act of bravery by queer individuals, it's just another part of who they are and it's treated by most people as just as important to their athletic lives as their shoe size or hair colour. You see this kind of attitude far more among younger people in Canada and North America, who have grown up with far more queer influences in their lives, especially in the mass media which has fostered a view that being queer is not something to be reviled, and is just something that's different. Therefore it's become something that younger generations are less concerned about as compared to their older peers, who may still hold to many of the stereotypes that grew out of the AIDS epidemic and the aftermath of that crisis.

Whole organizations are being developed to help create safe spaces for queer athletes to be who they are and compete at the highest levels of their sports, opening up new avenues for achievement in ways that just two decades ago felt like they were nearly impossible to fathom. In short, sports may be considered the final frontier and the last domain of accepted homophobia and transphobia, but even in the professional athletic world and the local community organizations that form the main interaction between people and athletics, those barriers are falling away and creating more inviting, inclusive spaces that accept and understand that a diverse membership that represents the entirety of their community is the best way to maintain strength and popularity for their sport.

There's no longer as much of a concern about what you are or how you identify when it comes to being part of professional or competitive athletics. The only thing that people are starting to care about is whether you can play the sport and contribute in a meaningful, positive way. This is being shown more and more as there are increasing numbers of athletes who are coming out and being told that it doesn't matter, they're still accepted because they play the sport better than people who could have been put on the team. That's the way it should be. Beyond this, there's also the greater societal acceptance of gays and lesbians that have been driving the willingness to allow more queer athletes to come out and be accepted. Rather than being seen as some invasion into something that's always been considered the territory of traditional masculinity, there's been a perceptive movement towards it being a matter of time before someone came out and played professionally, and that it's just how society is and how society should be that we can play at the highest levels of a sport.

Most importantly of all is that society itself seems okay with all these changes and is not trying overly hard to revert back to a society where queer individuals had to be in the closet to compete. There's no serious backlash against gays in sports or trans people in sports, and the most obvious concerns have been just that, concerns about how to properly integrate people into athletics without offending anyone or creating tense situations. These barriers aren't even being put up in the name of discrimination by most groups, and are grounded instead by a real misunderstanding of the issues at play; for trans athletes this is particularly true as there are a wider variety of concerns that need to be addressed for those who identify outside their biological sex than there would be for someone who has a minority sexual orientation. These are all things that are being changed one day at a time and that organizations and associations are learning to fix. That is the important thing, that we're now at a place and a time where these sports leagues want to make those changes because they know it's a benefit to themselves and their players, and that is something that wasn't true all that long ago.

Now that queer athletes are becoming more accepted in mainstream society and it's become easier for youth to see themselves reflected in their role models, there has been an increasing number of organizations devoted to providing support for these athletes or to create an environment in their league that would allow future athletes to feel comfortable enough to come out. The You Can Play Project is one of the best known of these organizations at this point in time, and is actively working with professional and collegiate teams to make their organizations more accepting and welcoming of queer athletes. You Can Play has more of a national and international focus, and as a result they have had more well-known sponsors and supporters of their organization. Their main goal is to provide training for teams to make their organizations more queer-friendly, but also to promote to youth of all ages and orientations that the only thing that should matter is the ability to play the game, and that your sexual orientation or gender identity are secondary to the ability to enjoy the sport.

Other local organizations may exist with similar purposes, depending on where you live and what kind of local environment already exists for queer athletes in your area. In Vancouver, the group Queer Active serves as a connector group, connecting queer youth with sports leagues that would be appropriate for them and also providing information about many of the queer-friendly or queer-only sports leagues that exist in the city and surrounding area. Queer Active in particular has started networking with local queer community centers to continue with their outreach and to ensure that as many people as possible are connected with leagues they are interested in. This would be an ideal place to check on the queer athletics situation in your own area, as these community centers are likely to either know about the situation themselves, or they will be able to connect you to one of the local organizations that should be working to provide safe queer athletics in the area.

Beyond these sorts of organizations there are also groups that have been active in the past to create more acceptance of queer athletics that may have had an impact in your area. During the early part of the century, the Fearless Campus Tour created an annual photo project of openly queer athletes in their natural athletic environment. The goal was to take these photographs and show that queer athletes are just as talented as their heterosexual comrades and to show that these athletes are everywhere. Attached to each athlete's set of photographs was information about where they played and the division of their sports, and it turned out that many of these athletes were openly queer and also playing at the highest levels of collegiate sports. The photo set would travel to different college campuses and highlight different athletes, and was even prominently displayed as part of the Vancouver Olympics Pride House, showing that even at the Olympic level there was growing acceptance of openly queer athletes.

The internet is becoming one of the fastest ways of spreading information between people, and it should come as no surprise that it's proving to be a vital gateway to sharing information about queer athletics. One of the best resources to be found on the web is the Outsports website, which tracks college and professional sports across North America. Their main purpose is to identify and help support queer athletes that are in the coming out process and to share their stories with other queer athletes, and they also provide information and stories about the professional athletic world that highlight cases where discrimination is being fought against. The site also includes a number of articles that do not discuss queer athletics and instead focus on upcoming events, such as the NCAA tournament and league championships, with significant analyses of the players and teams participating in those championships.

All of this information is great to have and it's wonderful to have resources available to teach queer athletes and coaches what to do when they get involved, but we're missing a crucial point here and that is to talk about how it is that we actually will manage to get ourselves involved in athletics at all, given the misconceptions that exist between queer people and the rest of society, misconceptions that are unfortunately found on both sides of the issue. For many queer athletes, the idea of participating in what would be considered mainstream leagues is unacceptable and would lead to a lot of extra emotional baggage that doesn't need to become part of the athletic experience. The number of queer people interested in participating in athletics has grown significantly in the last few years, and now there are organizations in many major cities in Canada that have their own listings of sports leagues that are welcoming to queer players regardless of skill level. These listings include a wide variety of sports and often have means of introducing new players to the leagues and ensuring that everyone is able to get along and that it serves as a good fit for people just starting out as athletes.

Vancouver has a clearinghouse of information regarding sports in the community and the near suburbs to the city itself through Queer Active, the organization that grew out of Team Vancouver. Queer Active focuses mainly on providing resources for queer youth who wish to become involved in athletics, but they also provide opportunities for people of all ages to become connected with queer-friendly sports leagues in the Metro Vancouver area. Queer Active includes information about seventeen different queerfriendly sports organization and a health organization that works closely with the queer community. Their website includes links to the websites of these leagues and associations, providing potential athletes with a single location in which they can find information about the sport of their choice. For those sports that do not have any queerfriendly league already associated with it or that Queer Active is aware of, they also offer the opportunity to be sponsored and gain funding and promotional opportunities to create your own queer-friendly league in a sport that is lacking queer representation in the city. This has meant that while there is already a vibrant queer sporting environment in Vancouver, there is always the potential for growth for people who want to take on the work needed to create new leagues.

Torontonians and those who live near Toronto are able to find information about queer-friendly sporting activities in their area through Outsports Toronto, which serves to highlight not just the organizations that are operating in the city and region, but also to highlight upcoming events that Outsports Toronto or its partner sporting leagues are hosting in the near future. Outsports Toronto includes information on thirty-three different organizations, and also includes links to those organizations websites for people to obtain additional information about those associations. Outsports includes additional information and resources that potential queer athletes and coaches will want to read and discuss before joining an athletic association, which is available to everyone who visits their website. Outsports Toronto is also a supporter of the gay games and gay olympics, and encourages people to participate in these athletic competitions as much as possible. This is something that both Queer Active in Vancouver and Equipe Montreal do as well, and appears to be common among all queer sporting associations that they promote these opportunities for international competition.

Equipe Montreal is the organization that works to ensure that members of the queer community in Montreal are able to get their athletic needs met. Their website is mainly written in French, as to better suit their local audience. Equipe Montreal has information about eighteen different organizations around the island that are accessible to queer athletes, and includes links to their websites as well as additional contact information for many of the groups. The organization also posts information and advertisements for events that their partner associations are promoting or hosting in the area. Unique to Equipe Montreal is that they have a monthly newsletter that they send to people who are on their mailing list which includes additional information about upcoming events and how to become more involved with the organization or any other organization that works with Equipe. The archives for this newsletter are kept on the organization's website and can be downloaded at any time, showing just how active the group has been and how involved they are in ensuring that there is a strong queer sports contingent out of Montreal.

A recent look through some of the major sports publications or news sites is talking about all the recent collegiate athletes who have come out of the closet, and the relative dearth of professional athletes who have done the same. It's worth discussing why those two different groups would have such different reactions and have far different coming out rates when they're generally all in the public eye, particularly in America where college athletics is a major industry and takes up a significant segment of the cultural mindset. Typical examples of this kind of thinking include Michigan stadium, better known as the Big House, which can seat over one hundred thousand people for its college football games, making it one of the largest fields in North America. This increased interest and scrutiny of college athletes in America makes it very similar to how professional sports are scrutinized and discussed in the media and among members of society, but there are far more queer college athletes than there are professional athletes. It would be nearly impossible to prove any one factor was the cause for the divergent figures, but there are certainly a number of possibilities that are worth discussing and addressing so that they can be better compensated for by groups attempting to create a safe environment for queer professional athletes.

The environment the players are involved in has to be one of the most important factors that goes into the decision to come out or not. We can generally accept that college campuses are among the more accepting places to be queer in North American society, with the majority of campuses having at least some kind of outreach center for queer students and faculty to meet with each other and provide support for one another. College campuses also have strong policies devoted to the protection of all their students and staff, which have recently been better and explicitly protecting members of the queer community. Once again using Michigan as an example, the University of Michigan banned a former assistant Attorney-General from their campus because of his campaign of homophobia and abuse towards one of its students, something that would not have been done even in recent memory. Even if one is to become part of the athletic scene in college, those individuals are first and foremost members of the university and subject to the values and beliefs of that school. More importantly, voluntarily joining these schools with strong policies and protections for queer people can be seen as at least an implicit endorsement of those same values by the student population, so there is less reason for queer athletes to fear a backlash when it's clear that there's at least an underlying acceptance of the idea of being tolerant and open towards those who are different.

This is contrasted with professional sports, where we have been led to believe the environment has been crafted to focus on extreme masculinity which has been defined as a strong focus on physical strength and heteronormativity among all members of the league or profession. In many cases this is supported through the personal beliefs of the professional athletes, which are often credited at least in part for the success of the athlete in achieving their professional dreams. What is created then is an environment where it is of social benefit to be aggressively masculine and devoted to the traditional family structure of a husband a wife with their children, which is what the fans, media and players themselves have been taught to believe is how professional athletics works, all told by the media that needs to maintain that kind of perspective for the purpose of sensationalizing those who do come out. Unfortunately, most people buy into this stereotyped view and perpetuate it for fear of losing sponsorships or contract money, which continue to be their means of funding during their careers and for a significant portion of their post-career lives.

This leads into the next factor, and that's the monetary difference between a professional and collegiate athlete. College athletes in both Canada and the United States are barred from accepting any kind of salary or compensation in exchange for their playing abilities. This is skirted around a little with the ability for NCAA schools to offer sports scholarships that cover the entire costs of education for the student, but in terms of actual contracts or benefits the students are not paid to play. Student-athletes don't have to worry about losing sponsorship deals or contract bonuses or anything else other than playing their sport and focusing on their academics, which is how it should be given that they are still students at their school.

By comparison, professional athletes by their very definition derive their income from their work, and thus anything that could possibly reduce or eliminate their ability to play and get sponsorships and endorsements is something that needs to be either minimized or eliminated entirely. The prevailing view among most professional athletes seems to be that it would be alright to have a queer teammates and it wouldn't' cause a problem, but most are genuinely unsure of how that teammate would perform or how their contracts would be affected by coming out. This is mostly because of the concern, especially for star players, that the fans would stop supporting that player of their team and reduce team revenues, which eventually cuts into the salaries of the players themselves. Endorsements might also become harder for professional athletes to obtain from corporate sponsors who are unwilling to potentially alienate any of their clients. All of this radiates from the media viewpoint that tells society that professional athletics is entirely heteronormative and that it is not ready for queer players yet.

The media exerts a huge influence on all of society and the perceptions we have about our societal institutions. It should come as no surprise that the media also influences the way we think about athletics and athletes. In the case of athletics, the media has been continuously saying that professional sports and even collegiate sports are not ready for the circus that will erupt should a player actually come out. Left unsaid is the fact that media itself is creating the circus that they fear will happen whenever an athlete comes out.

The idea of professional athletes admitting and publicly stating that they are queer is nothing new. We have had queer players in our national sports leagues for decades now, and more often than not it's met with a collective shrug by the fans, and only a few days of media coverage. That's because up until this past year, the only professional athletes who have come out of the closet were retired and had nothing to lose by being free about who they are. Athletes like Billy Bean were astounding us with their skills on the field long before anyone thought that they should come out and say who they were, and as it turns out people weren't all that interested when they did come out because their day was over. They were retired athletes and while it was interesting to reflect on how they must have felt living in a homophobic work environment, they weren't there anymore and no one really had to think about how their behaviour was affecting someone that they played with right then and there.

The truth of the matter is that it revolved around money, and it still does to a certain degree. Professional athletes derive their livelihood and their ability to earn a living from their sport, and up until recently they had no reason to assume that they would be considered welcome after they came out. Coaches, fans, the media and even other players would routinely make statements about how they would have problems playing with an openly gay player and how it would present problems for both the team and for the individual who chooses to come out. Some players have even indicated that it would put an openly queer player in physical danger as other players attempt to harm them in response to being out. Then there is the consideration of whether an openly queer player could get signed, based on these fears and the considerations that coaches would have to take into account when signing players that might become liabilities either because of their own play or how they distract the rest of the team.

The most important issue that would be considered by queer athletes deciding whether to come out would have been and likely continues to be whether they will continue to get contracts and be able to play. The viability of queer athletes has been questioned regularly since it became a potential issue, with players from multiple sports indicating that it would be problematic for people to be openly queer and still want to consider an athletics career. This viewpoint is shared by some coaches and has led to some coaches being forced into sensitivity training to ensure they refrain from making discriminatory comments in the future. It would be fairly safe to say that most players' agents are aware of these underlying feelings and may even share them, which would complicate the ability for a player to be given a fair opportunity to get a playing contract with a team, even for a minor league deal. While it would have been of greater concern a few decades ago, recent experiences have shown that there still remains difficulties for queer athletes to be taken seriously and that it could potentially lead to a lack of ability to get signed. In 2001, Leigh Steinberg, a sports agent, noted that he thought 'it would have a devastating effect in terms of the marketability of any athlete to come out and talk about gayness', highlighting concerns in the athletic community about the ability for players to bring in sales and ensure they can contribute financially to the organization. It's disappointing that there needs to be a financial consideration taken when it should be about hiring the best player for the team, but sports teams are corporations and they do need to ensure a profit for themselves and their ownership group. This means that even now there may be some apprehension about the ability for queer players to be signed and added to a team's roster.

The issue of locker room acceptance continues to be a problem for queer athletes around the world, but in professional sports it becomes a matter of greater urgency given that these athletes are bound to play with each other through a contract and that it provides a livelihood for those who are able to participate. It's always good to participate in recreational athletics and I would hope all queer athletes are able to do so, but when it becomes a matter of how you pay the rent and your other expenses it evolves into a matter of ensuring that your workplace is not actively discriminatory against you. The United States currently has no national protection against workplace discrimination, which includes the locker rooms of our professional sports leagues. This means that it is perfectly legal for a team or organization to discriminate against openly queer players and refuse to sign them on the grounds that they are gay. Which isn't to say that it wouldn't happen if there was an anti-discrimination law in effect, there are always reasons to avoid signing someone, but for a queer player at least it would give them some recourse should they face discrimination once signed to a team and they began upholding their part of the player's contract. Without those protections many players have gone on the record talking about how they are not accepting of queer people in general and more specifically about the possibility of queer people playing on their teams. Society and professional sports have gotten better at addressing these kinds of comments in recent years, but they still happen often enough that they would present a formidable barrier and justification for remaining in the closet during the course of one's career.

Even assuming that a player can be signed, his or her marketability or ability to ensure profits for their team is constantly being questioned, and queer players or players who are perceived to be queer are put through more scrutiny than their heterosexual teammates. In 2013 during the controversy surrounding Manti Te'o, it was learned that many of the college athletes at the NFL scouting combine were asked questions about their sexual orientation or their personal lives that were deemed to be of no influence to their ability to play football, but were considered part of the scouting combine and had to be answered by the potential players. Earlier this year after Michael Sam came out as a gay college athlete, it was believed by many scouts and the media that his ability to be drafted would suffer because of his decision to come out. His playing ability had not been affected by the decision, but it was still seen as a potential liability in the world of professional athletics and was thus seen as downgrading his 'stock' as a potential candidate for the draft. Lower draft numbers generally correlate with lower overall salaries and a reduced ability to gain the playing time needed to secure longer term contracts in the future, so this perception of homosexuality as a negative attribute in professional athletics could negatively affect players' ability to earn a salary. The other main consideration with regards to the personal finances of the player is their ability to be marketed and endorsed for products, which increases the visibility of the player and the team that they play for. Corporate sponsorships constitute a significant income source independent of the player's contract with their team, and many players endorse products that have nothing to do with their sport in order to gain those additional sources of income. For corporations concerned about the perception of being associated with a queer athlete, this historically was cause for concern and made corporations shy away from athletes that could potentially be considered queer and back towards 'safer' athletes who would not upset key marketing demographic. Current polling indicates that there are growing majorities of people in North America who are supportive of queer people, but whether that extends specifically to the demographics of individuals most likely to purchase sports apparel or other products that are often endorsed by professional athletes has not been tested, and would serve as a final concern for athletes who may consider coming out.

Beyond the monetary concerns and the ability to actually play the sport they love, closeted queer athletes also have to consider if they want to deal with the media attention of being one of the first people to come out in professional sports. Jason Collins is currently the only professional basketball player who has come out of the closet, and he is currently in his first year of playing professionally. In spite of his inexperience and how new he is to the league, the media pays a significant amount of attention to him and his activities, and he remains a controversial figure whenever he plays. This kind of media attention, rightly called a media circus by those who are forced to endure it, distracts from the ability to play the sport and constitutes the very distractions that coaches and agents often fear will occur when dealing with potential controversy. Michael Sam has not yet even been drafted into the NFL and there are already media crews that focus on him and what he will mean to the NFL and to America more generally because he's already out of the closet. Neither gentleman asked to become a mascot or anything other than a professional athlete, and to try and force them to be representative of those who are not yet out forces them into a precarious media situation where they are forced into being spokespeople for a whole segment of society. Because of the usually unwanted nature of these kinds of inquisitions into the lives of queer athletes and the intense media coverage that has occurred for those few who have come out, other queer athletes will have to consider whether they are willing to have that same level of media scrutiny placed upon them for the foreseeable future as the media decides to devote its energy to determining how they would serve as some kind of message for North America, and this only serves to take away from the point that queer athletes are trying to make; that we're there to play the sport and succeed in the athletic component of the game, as opposed to trying to be a societal message. That the media itself often does not understand that makes it more difficult for the message to come across, and may serve to eliminate the willingness for other players to come out themselves.

It's become clear that most of the concerns about coming out in professional sports is based around each player and each team's bottom line, and that there needs to be a degree of respect for the personal privacy of the players who do choose to come out. These are fundamental issues that need to be addressed and it remains to be seen how individual people can do so and have the effect needed to persuade other athletes to come out. This is particularly true with regards to the need for personal privacy; our national and local media seem incapable of not delving into stories that are based around people's personal lives and digging to see what kind of scandals can be found, and that can't be controlled by anyone except the reporters themselves, and they seem far more interested in getting the scoop than doing what's right and dignified for the subject of their numerous articles.

The media is the most difficult variable to control when it comes to showing support for queer athletes who are thinking of coming out, and paradoxically the answer to creating a situation where it becomes safe for athletes to come out is to simply ignore them when it happens. Our instincts are always to pay attention to the issue because it is something that's novel and unexpected among our national athletes and our college athletes. We think of them as nothing but a pack of heterosexual men and women, and anything else seriously interrupts our stereotypes and assumptions about what it means to be a professional athlete. It means that we as a society and culture can do nothing but to gawk and stare at someone who is different, and the media realizes that this is a story they can use to gain more attention for themselves. It's often said among media types that if it bleeds, it leads, and that was always put forward as the justification for putting particularly violent episodes or other events that are bound to grab our attention as the first thing shown during a newscast. The reason always being that the first few minutes or the front pages are when people are most interested and tuned in, and as the news goes on people become less interested in what's being said, so there's a need to instantly grab the viewer's attention with something unexpected or traumatic that will be remembered and retain viewership in the future. If we as a society start denying that to media outlets in their coverage of athletes who come out, the outlets themselves will conclude that there's no need for hyperventilating or exaggerated coverage, and they'll find something else to take the lead, which will help free athletes from having to deal with constant media scrutiny about their personal lives.

The rest of it is within our power to do, and indeed where there have been openly queer athletes the results have been astounding at the level of public support they have received. In the weeks since Jason Collins was signed by the New Jersey Nets basketball team, sales of their merchandise has increased, and the sales of Collins branded merchandise became the most popular selling item among all merchandise sold by any NBA franchise for over a week. Fans have taken to going to games where he is scheduled to play even when New Jersey is the visiting team, simply to show their support for having an openly gay basketball player that is able to compete on an equal footing with his heterosexual peers. In terms of creating a market and affecting the bottom line profits of the team, it would appear that Jason Collins has been a huge benefit not just to his own team but everywhere he goes he seems to be increasing ticket sales, and that can only lead to additional sales of other goods and merchandise while those people are at a game. This isn't something that was done consciously by the teams to ensure a good marketing rollout, that was done by everyday fans showing up and voting with their wallets about how comfortable they felt with a player who so obviously defied what it meant to be an athlete. It doesn't feel like it when you're buying a t-shirt or a jersey with Collins' name on it or watching Johnny Weir on tv, but sports teams look at those trends and they start feeling less concerned about queer athletes hurting their bottom line and damaging the financial viability of their businesses.

As for the players themselves, they're sure to know what it is that is bringing people out, and are likely to understand that it helps their brand to be known as someone who is able to move merchandise; like any other consumer good branding is important and having a good brand is worth a fair bit. It shouldn't be in sports, since the only thing that should matter is your ability to play the sport, but for professional teams who are always looking to increase their revenues and professional athletes who are looking to sign better contracts, it helps to be able to prove they can deliver, and so far Jason Collins has been able to do so. It remains to be seen how stable that will be, though his ability to keep playing well should help with that regard, but it does get noticed by other players. This also gets noticed by outside organizations and corporations who are interested in partnering with endorsement deals. It hasn't happened yet, but it wouldn't be surprising to see Jason Collins or other prominent queer athletes like Tom Daley of Great Britain get a significant endorsement deal because of how high profile they have become as part of their coming out process. Relating this to the bottom line for queer athletes is simple; this is more money they have and it makes a difference by showing that there won't be negative fallout from coming out, and that the only major consequence will be freeing themselves from the burden of having to hide or lie about who they are as a person.

These options remain available to most sports teams and organizations, but very few commit to doing so. The honest reason that many of these sports teams don't get involved with explicitly queer advertising or making direct overtures to queer fans is that no one has asked them to before, and they don't know what the market is going to be like where they live. There are always some owners and managers who are going to be opposed for their own personal reasons, and those are more often found in culturally conservative parts of North America, but the vast majority of organizations are going to be concerned solely with earning more money for themselves, however that is best able to be done.

This is where community leadership is key. Sports teams may not normally go out of their way to create specific queer advertising, but they're more than willing to sell the tickets if people in the community are willing to do the legwork needed to advertise and ensure that there will be a group of people ready to buy those tickets. Many sports teams, especially in major league baseball, have taken to having specific 'gay day' events where a significant segment of the population in the stands identifies as part of the queer community. These events are not the idea of the sports teams, but are actually pitched to the teams by community leaders who then make sure they can find people to fill the seats. These events have become increasingly popular both within sports and outside of sports, with Disneyworld having an annual gay day event that is hosted through the creation of a full-time position dedicated to ensuring the event is well-attended. Disneyworld can do that, but most sports teams do not have the manpower available to do the advertising and run these events themselves, even if they were interested in doing so, as the Toronto Blue Jays were.

For teams that embrace these sorts of events that highlight support for the queer community and its inclusion in athletics, there's a good reason why they continue to happen each and every year after the initial event; they work. Outside of a few major rivalry games, it's pretty hard to sell out a stadium each and every home game, and having a group come in and say they'd like to buy a certain number of tickets that the team is already having difficulty selling makes a great deal of economic sense to the teams. Most teams are also situated in relatively urban areas, and recent polling has shown that in North America, areas of greater urban density have been more supportive of queer rights, so highlighting support for a significant part of the local community serves to benefit the team and is not often seen as going against the cultural grain of their community. This level of support also means that with additional people in the seats, more merchandise is being sold and more profits are being made by the team.

The only disappointing part is that right now, for all the success that has occurred with these gay day events, they're still mostly run by the community organizations that have been proposing them to start, and the teams just passively collect the benefits of additional revenues without doing anything to stimulate further growth from the queer community. There's a growing amount of outreach from gay and lesbian organizations into organized athletics, and what needs to start happening is a reciprocal amount of outreach from the teams who are benefiting from these gay days and have them start reaching out into their local queer communities to see how they can repay some of that kindness.

For one thing, it just makes sense; by showing an active interest in a growing market and segment of the population that wants to be part of the team's fanbase, these teams can start showing they care about more than just the money and create genuine links in the community that will make more queer people feel welcome at sports events. At this point in history it shouldn't be, but it would also be a sign that the era of overt homophobia in society was at an end if professional sports teams and organizations were to make concerted efforts to court queer people and have them become an integral part of what athletics in North America looks like. Too often the assumption and marketing strategies are based on younger heterosexual males and the people they often bring with them to games; families and their friends or girlfriends. It's worked so far, but creating more inclusive outreach strategies would be seen at this point in time as a bold step and signal that discrimination is not acceptable and that there's no obvious demographic that would be more or less interested in sports, which would go a long way to reducing the prevalence of the stereotype that queer people are not interested in sports at all.

The solutions that have been proposed by the research are admirable and will likely have a positive effect on the locker room environment and in reducing homophobia and transphobia in athletics, but more needs to be done to ensure that these practices are changed on a uniform basis within all organizations. Too often these kinds of minor changes by having more out athletes only creates change within one or two individuals or teams within an organization. In the context of the athletic world, this is too small of a change to be considered a true success, particularly for those youth who aren't fortunate enough to be part of those teams and thus would have to deal with the same kinds of discrimination that they have always had to address. Which isn't to say that we shouldn't commit to those kinds of reforms and those policies that have been described in the research and have widespread support; if having more out athletes and publicizing that they are out and still able to participate in athletics helps even one person become more accepted for who they are among their peers, then it should be considered a successful policy that has done what it needed to do. This is becoming more tenable as a potential policy change, as there are increasing numbers of athletes who are well known and who are coming out. Even if that was to suddenly end in the next few days and weeks, there would still be a large number of examples that coaches and parents could point to and say that these people are successful athletes who happen to have a queer identity, which is a better position than just a few years ago when it was almost impossible to name an openly queer athlete who was still actively playing their sport.

This also is an issue of concern with regards to the creation of queer-friendly leagues. These leagues would have specific policies put into place that would allow for queer athletes to participate without having to fear that they will be the target of discriminatory actions, but this will also have the negative effect of reducing the need for mainstreamed leagues to create their own policies and instead assume that the entirety of their membership will be made of heterosexual and cisgendered participants. In doing so, this lack of motivation will ensure that these leagues remain segregated and will create the aforementioned problems for queer athletes who seek to participate at elite or competitive levels that may not be available to them in casual queer leagues. Within the queer friendly leagues themselves this could be addressed by having different skill level groups if the numbers allow for that kind of division, but that also would tend to perpetuate the idea of segregation being the final solution for queer athletes who want to participate in athletics. This difficulty in balancing the need to create a safe space for queer athletes to participate and meet other queer athletes needs to be considered alongside the needs of some of those same players to have a space where they will be able to compete and mature as players, hopefully to the point where they are able to participate in the level of competition they are hoping to reach in their athletics careers. What could be done, assuming there was a willingness from both sides, would be to have some kind of crossover tournament or competition where teams from both the specifically queer-friendly league and the more mainstream leagues would be able to compete against each other and see that there were skilled players on both sides of the equation. Doing so would help reduce the fear and concern that straight athletes would have about participating with queer athletes, and queer athletes would have an opportunity to compete against different teams or players who are of a different calibre than what they are used to coming from the queer friendly leagues. Eventually, as these kinds of cooperative events become more common and there becomes more understanding and opportunities for learning between different leagues, there may become less of a need for having specifically queer friendly leagues as a safe space. These sorts of leagues are still likely to exist even after openly queer men and women become accepted in mainstream athletics because it will still create an opportunity to meet other queer people, so the risk of these leagues losing the entirety of their membership is quite low.

The answer that I feel is most likely to create sustainable benefits and allow for more queer people to feel that they are welcome in athletics of all levels is to create dedicated policies at each of the leagues, or preferably at the level of the provincial sporting authority that creates clear guidelines on participation and behaviour, which should have as its basis the need for all participants to feel welcome and to outline specifically how discrimination should be addressed by the members of that organization or league. The main reason for a league or provincial policy would be to ensure uniformity and create opportunities for all individuals to play, even in areas that would otherwise be more hostile than areas of Canada that have large queer populations and greater support for the queer community. This is where the main concern would be; there are already many sports groups in urban areas that already have policies protecting queer participants because there's a higher concentration of queer people who live in those areas. Queer people who live in places like Vancouver, Toronto or Montreal and already enjoy significant protections in terms of their ability to live their lives without outward discrimination are fine, but there are still many areas of Canada where it can be difficult to be openly queer, and it is those areas that would need the protection of a policy that is created at the provincial level and that could be enforced on organizations to ensure protections are put in place and adhered to during the season. Rather than leaving each organization to create their own rules and to create a patchwork of different policies that have different overall impacts and levels of effectiveness in protecting queer and heterosexual athletes, a single policy adopted by all sports organizations in a province or jurisdiction would ensure that everyone is on the same wavelength and has the same understanding of what is acceptable. This allows youth participants to ensure that they can participate in a location that is suitable for them based on their athletic needs, instead of having to travel greater distances to ensure they participate in a program that offers protections to them.

There have been very few past policy changes at the grassroots level regarding the need to address homophobic bullying or any kind of discrimination within youth sports. The general policy has been for the athletes themselves to work out their differences, with the coaches or parents intervening only when it becomes clear that the participants are unable to conclude the issue on their own. This is something that I have noticed quite consistently through my own sporting career, in that none of my coaches felt comfortable getting involved in the bullying behaviour of the players unless it became clear that the issue was going to devolve into a fight or other situation that would be seen as an escalation from typical youth behaviour and into actions that could cause serious harm to the athletes. This often meant that the behaviour would continue until the player fought back, which often ended poorly for that player, given they were often targeted for the same reason that any other child is bullied; because they're weaker or seen as weaker and less able to respond effectively to the bullying that was occurring. When it came to me, I was chosen as a target specifically because of assumptions about my low weight and slight physical frame, which was perceived to be physically weaker than my peers on the team. There was also a perception that I would not respond violently or that the aggressive players would be able to handle my response, which is often associated with bullying. The overall result was that the bullying would continue unopposed by anyone, and my lack of response was considered to be consent for it to continue. All of these assumptions were accepted as normal by the coaching staff and the rest of the team, and thus there was nothing done to address the concerns, in spite of how they were negatively affecting me and hampering my ability to remain competitive. A lot of this occurred because the coaches themselves hadn't been given adequate training into the effects of discriminatory language in athletics and how they affect players, and so they felt it was just juvenile behaviour that they could safely ignore.

This lack of consistent or coherent policy development for how to intervene and protect athletes from homophobic or transphobic discrimination is further exacerbated by the fact that there appears to be no required training that addresses these kinds of issues in sports. Neither the players nor the coaches have to undergo any kind of training regarding issues of discrimination, which often means that such interventions are left to the personal opinions and beliefs of the coach or parents. This can create situations where the administration of any policies that do exist may become unfair or irregularly administered, or simply ignored based on the feelings of the coach and their beliefs about what is happening to their players. There's no reason to believe that it's always or even predominantly based on coaches having prejudices against queer people, but there remains a consistent view among coaches that there are specific attitudes and beliefs that are considered acceptable in the athletic world and that they won't attempt to intervene against because they're seen as ways of building camaraderie or character in the players that are suffering, and that they will end up being better players and better people because of it. There's no evidence to support that notion, but it has become a part of the conventional wisdom surrounding sports that there needs to be some kind of hazing done to toughen up the players and ensure that they are able to survive in athletics, which are often quite physical and based on traditionally masculine ideals, such as aggression and dominance over others. These traits are found even in women's sports, where there remains a need to stay competitive and to defeat the opposing team or player. Where they occur in women's sports they also bring into play a degree of sexism that requires female players to take on traits that are traditionally identified as masculine and to shed some of their femininity in order to remain competitive. This view that there must be a sacrifice of some of the traits that players may naturally identify with in order to be accepted by the group is it's own form of discrimination, with the forced uniformity of the personalities of the players creating a situation where retaining those differences, and in this case specifically a queer identity that runs counter to stereotypes of those traits that are considered acceptable in athletics, leading to ostracism and reduced outcomes for the players that are discriminated against.

This can be solved through the creation of two province-wide or national policies that would apply equally to all sports organizations; one that specifically prohibits discrimination of any participant on any protected ground in the Canadian Constitution, and a second policy requiring that coaches undergo diversity training that would give them the tools to properly address any situation that may arise in the course of their duties as coaches and guardians of children. With regards to the policy idea of creating a clause in every sports organization's charter stating that all forms of discrimination should be banned in their league, this is meant to ensure that the local grassroots understand that there will be zero tolerance for any form of discrimination. By specifically naming the forms of discrimination that are to be opposed and considered unacceptable, it makes clear to participants and their parents that this change in policy is accepted by the league and the organization, and that staying as part of the league will require adhering to those points of view. It's a clear statement in favour of protecting the rights of queer youth from being discriminated against. These sorts of policies also already exist with a number of different organizations outside of sports, and they continue to have high levels of participation and the support of their communities. Examples include the Canada Boy Scouts, which have a firm policy rejecting discrimination of any kind from among their troops and separates them from their more well-known American counterparts. The Boy Scouts continue to have very high membership rates in spite of having these policies in place, and indeed there are reasons to believe that having these strong membership policies that protect the safety of all members positively contribute to the ability of these organizations to maintain and expand their memberships. Policies requiring coaches to undergo specific diversity training to ensure they understand the needs of the diverse groups of players they may encounter as coaches may be more difficult to achieve, particularly if that kind of programming remains outside the requirements of coaching certification and would not be considered part of the traditional coaching certification process. Having an incentive of some kind for coaches that voluntarily complete this kind of training would be helpful, as would having some kind of support in place to recuperate the financial costs of these kinds of diversity training programs, particularly with regards to parents who decide to coach and may not have the means or time to spend in additional theoretical work when they simply want to coach their child's team. Creating partnerships with organizations that deliver diversity training and incorporating those groups into the sports association would be another way in which coaches could obtain the information they need without having to create too much of an additional cost for potential coaches. This would be more likely to be effective than to have a generalized coaching course add diversity issues into a program that already attempts to put too much into too short a time period to adequately prepare coaches for their teams and the process of playing.

We already have separate policies put in place requiring prospective coaches to undergo police investigations and other training that is deemed to be important to the growth of the sport and protection of children, and some of those courses cover ethics and other issues relevant to the needs of coaching. There should be no problem including a course that includes issues of diversity, particularly if it covers other areas of potential discrimination that may occur in the course of athletics. While it is likely that there will be complaints from some coaches that they will be required to participate in training that runs contrary to their personal beliefs, it is important to remember that more is at stake than the personal beliefs of the coaching staff of youth athletics; the role of the coach is to serve as a mentor and leader for their team, and that cannot be done while actively or passively discriminating against members of their team. The goal of this change in coaching policy to require diversity training will be to inform coaches of their potential biases and ensure that they have the personal understanding to ensure that they do not create situations where they discriminate against any of their players.

The biggest concern with the creation of wholesale policy changes is the difficulty in obtaining the sustained attention of policy makers and important stakeholders in any final decision that has to be made about those impending policy changes. The general consensus for policy makers and administrators is that the system they have created is already acceptable because it is stable and there are no reports of any extreme behaviour to attract their attention. As long as the issues of discrimination are being unreported or reported as minor instances, those in charge of dictating and creating policy in athletics organizations are unlikely to intervene. This is particularly true of sports, where a certain amount of aggression is expected, to the point where commentary that would be considered vulgar and discriminatory in civil society would be considered tolerated in the context of athletics. This unfortunately means that in many cases where there are legitimate concerns about discrimination, there is an unwillingness to fully investigate the claims or concerns because it is assumed to be part of the athletic experience.

Meeting with these administrators and board directors becomes one of the first steps that must be done once it becomes determined that a policy change is required and that no other solution will work to make your organization safe for all players. However, for the most part the leaders of these organizations are not always easy to find, and even if you can find one or two members of the board that you need to speak to, it becomes very difficult for people to actually accomplish anything due to how infrequently the boards meet to discuss matters of the association. Bringing the issue up at the annual general meeting of the association is unlikely to be acceptable either, as the likely response will be to push the issue off until the following annual general meeting the next year, as they won't have had time to discuss the issue and would prefer for the next year's group of board members to deal with the issue instead of dealing with it immediately prior to the elections for board of directors. The recommended means of ensuring that the policy change is placed on the association's agenda is to speak with those members of the association that you can, when you can, and keep in communication with them until the annual general meeting comes up. Providing the incumbent board members with information showing why you think it is important for this kind of discussion to take place will also help keep the issue foremost on the minds of the association board members, and gives them some information they can use once they are at the meeting that can help make the process smoother and quicker.

This means that it becomes incumbent upon the athletes or their guardians to initiate claims of discrimination or inform their organization of any kind of discrimination. For young players who have already been abused by their teammates or opponents, it is a terrifying thought to have to tell someone else about what has transpired, particularly when it is clear that very little has been done in the past to address those concerns. In most cases, the athlete being discriminated against will simply withdraw the complaint, or as is the case with most athletes, they simply won't make the complaint to begin with. This ends up contributing to the overall view of the organization's administrators that there is no need for a policy change. However, this is just masking the fact that there are complaints being made, and that it is the forum itself that is making it difficult for the players to actively take part and explain what the problem is. There's also an inherent shame factor at having to admit to being discriminated against and not being able to solve the problem on their own, which is once again especially true for younger players, who may feel as though they're letting themselves be hurt by a bully when the response should be to either ignore them or to deal with the abuse in another way. For these kinds of situations it is helpful to collect information from all the complaints of discrimination made and to create some kind of information package that shows just how many players have made complaints about discrimination, and how that has changed over the past few years of the organization. Having concrete numbers crystallizes the issue in the minds of the people who are going to be making the final decision, and also means that those who have been discriminated against do not have to initially come forward and explain their stories. Eventually, however, it would be helpful to have those players come forward to the board and explain what actually happened when they were discriminated against, both to increase the emotional impact of the argument in favour of a policy change but also so that the policy makers can determine the best way of addressing the specific problems that occurred. This is something that would have to be agreed upon by the board of directors, your group of people helping to create the policy change and the players themselves. Asking for a venue that isn't as crowded or oppositional as an annual general meeting is a good idea, and in particular having a committee work on the issue that can report back to the board later creates an environment that is less oppositional and more inquisitive and is focused on finding the truth, and may be safer for players to come forward and express their concerns.

It is also difficult to simply have the league organizers show up at a game or practice and see for themselves what is being done and how much of a need there is for a policy change. In many situations in youth athletics, even if the players do not know who the new person is that is watching them, the coaches often do and are more likely to enforce rules or present their team in the best possible light, so as to avoid any potential punishment from the league organizers or officials. This often means that if informal checks are made to identify the extent of homophobic or transphobic discrimination, the administrators are left with the impression that there is no problem and any concerns are being exaggerated in order to promote an agenda. This is particularly difficult to dispel when it conforms to the views of the administrators. The solution to this kind of administrative resistance from policymakers is to provide detailed accounts of what is happening at the participant level and have those experiences be documented. Presenting those views to the appropriate body is an incredibly effective means of explaining to those in charge of sports programs that they need to act, especially when done at a public venue such as one of their general meetings, where any member of the league can speak and participate.

When we set out to create policy 5.45 and ensure that homophobic and transphobic discrimination would not be permitted in our schools in Burnaby, it became pretty clear that we would have to address a singular question that would be on everyone's minds; how would this help more than just the people it is meant to target? Better phrased, how would creating a new policy designed to help LGBTQ students also help out students who didn't identify as part of the queer community? It's a bit of an unusual question, since it should be clear that helping prevent discrimination against queer students was a good enough reason to act, particularly with the statistics that are routinely delivered showing just how much worse off queer students are compared to their non-queer peers. However, it is something we looked at and we found that it wasn't just queer students who were being discriminated against and who had homophobic or transphobic language used against them; it was everyone. It's been a long time since there was any kind of study or research done that showed that heterosexual students were totally immune to any form of homophobic or transphobic abuse, which seemed to highlight the fact that these kinds of abuses were far more common than anyone seemed to think.

We decided to change the way we pursued the policy change and instead looked at how our new policy would bring about changes that would positively affect the rest of the community, and we found that it was far easier to get the attention of policy makers once they were aware of how the change could be made to help everyone instead of just a single minority within the overall population. In the case of policy 5.45, we talked a lot about how student self-esteem was lowered when subjected to homophobic language, even for those who did not identify as queer or in the queer community. This gave us an opportunity to say that blanket changes would have the potential effect of ensuring that students were made safe who we already assumed considered themselves safe at our schools, and indeed the new policy is quite clear that it is the language used that is of concern and would be addressed, not who it targeted.

This is the key goal of any potential attempt to change policy within an organization, especially a sports organization that may not have anti-discrimination policies at the top of their agenda. Policy change is difficult at the best of times when it's clear that the change in question will have a positive impact on all or most members of the organization. What is more difficult still is the prospect of creating policy changes that appear to have an effect on only a small group of people within the larger organization and to do so without creating feelings of frustration and alienation within the organization towards the group that is proposing the policy change. These feelings of alienation occur most often when members of the majority group in the organization feel that they are being asked to give up rights or power in order to protect or promote a minority group. This has been recorded in society already with attitudes towards affirmative action programs, which are sometimes seen as favouring one minority group over the rest of society.

When creating large-scale policy changes, it is important to ensure that everyone feels that they are being positively affected by the change and that it is not meant to create a situation similar to the affirmative action feelings that occur in those who feel as though they are most vulnerable to any incoming change. This can be done by highlighting with evidence how the incoming change actually affects those groups in the organization positively and will not create any of the negative consequences that are feared by groups that oppose the changes being proposed. This often means that individuals who are interested in pursuing a policy change within their organization have to do research to ensure that there are unlikely to be negative consequences to the actions being proposed and also to be knowledgeable enough to answer any questions that other members of the organization may have about what is being proposed.

Changing local and organizational policies to create more queer-friendly teams and places where queer youth can participate in the same activities as their peers without fearing discrimination or harm has obvious benefits to the youth who are directly affected by the change in policy, but there are also benefits to those who are not going to be directly affected by any policy change. As the research has shown, even those who identify as heterosexual are targeted with homophobic and transphobic slurs or discriminatory action. These youth have also reported that the level of abuse they face, even though they are secure in their own sexuality, was often enough to make them reconsider staying as part of an organized athletic group. For organizations trying to maintain a strong membership base, finding ways to fight discrimination not only ensures a queer membership group but also ensures that the heterosexual membership does not feel alienated into leaving as well.

Returning to the idea of ensuring that there is effective buy-in from the rest of the organization, individuals who wish to try and create queer-friendly policies in their organization should look to see what has been done in other leagues and groups, if there are any in your local area. Most teams and leagues are willing to talk about how new policies have worked with regards to ending discrimination or other concerns that may be felt by their members, and having that additional information available when coming to make changes in your own teams is vital to alleviating concerns about how the process will play out. This is especially true if the policy change is expected to have a large impact or deviates significantly from past practice; knowing that other groups are beginning or have already done similar policy changes and have not been negatively affected by those changes will help reduce tension and fear about how the creation of queer-friendly policies will affect your own organization.

With many organizations, even if there is interest in creating policies that are going to help reduce discrimination against queer youth, there may be a lack of expertise and understanding of how to do that. This is a prime opportunity to seek partners from the community or beyond who have the expertise needed and are interested in working with your sports organization to create clear-cut policies that will have the intended effect of reducing discriminatory bullying in your league. Boards of directors will appreciate knowing they have the option of receiving help from these outside groups because it reduces the stress of the policy change process and demonstrates that other groups beyond the immediately affected youth are willing to pursue the kinds of policy ideas that are likely to be needed to create safe environments for all participants to enjoy. The groups you will want to talk to about working with your sports organizations are also normally quite happy to get involved and help where they can, all that's really needed is someone to approach them and say that there's a need for your sports organization to be given more information about how to become more queer-friendly and they will be happy to accommodate you.

There are few reasons to avoid working with other organizations when trying to create a more positive experience for the youth in any organization. Potential partners will have experiences and ideas for how to make your organization better managed or more accessible to potential participants and they also provide a new perspective on what's already working. The opportunity to trade information and create a series of best practices for the teams themselves often creates opportunities to make the league more responsive to the needs of the youth in general. Most importantly, most of these potential partner organizations have useful information on the technical aspect of the sports themselves, so partnering with queer sports organizations provides another set of coaches to help teach young players the fundamentals of the sport and will improve their athletic abilities, as well as providing a new perspective on some of their potential teammates and creating a safer environment for all players.

While there are doubtless going to be a large number of organizations that you can partner with to provide information to the league you are a member of in order to create safer spaces for queer athletes to participate, there needs to be a bit of research done by you and the rest of the people who are hoping for a policy change before anyone brings the idea to the league's board of directors. Have a look at the organization and see what kind of track record they have in working with other sports organizations in your city. Don't be afraid to expand beyond the city you live in either, especially if you find that there aren't that many organizations that look like they could be helpful to you. There are a number of national organizations in both Canada and the United States that are working to eliminate discriminatory barriers in athletics, and a fair number of them work on queer athletics issues as well. Many of these groups will also have greater resources and could be able to travel to your location if it became necessary. It also depends on what the specific issue is that has to be addressed; some organizations, such as You Can Play, are great when it comes to promoting the idea that sexual orientation and gender identity should not matter when participating in sports, and that it should be the skill of the player that is most important. That's great, but it may not address the specific issue that your organization is having, and you may find that it's more helpful to go to more specific organizations who have more information about your problem. As an example, there are likely to be groups run by trans activists who would have more information on how to create safe changing room spaces for trans athletes, something that is a continual concern of players both cisgendered and transgendered, and is currently one of the main barriers to participation for trans athletes.

In addition to providing coaching and other material gains for your youth, these organizations such as the You Can Play Project or Queer Active in Vancouver can also inform youth about other sports that have queer-friendly organizations or policies that your organization can learn from in terms of creating policies that will be of benefit to participants, without worrying that the alternative leagues are going to poach participants and reduce the number of members the organization has in future years. These organizations understand that sports associations survive through the continued participation of their members and will be happy to help work with your association to ensure that all members are eager to return in future years and do not feel that they have been ignored either during the policy creation or implementation phase of the new policies to protect queer youth.

The only major concern associated with working with these kinds of outside groups is that they will often have some kind of fee or honourarium that they will want to obtain from the organization for their services. This isn't exactly going to come as a surprise to anyone; they're providing a service and should be compensated for it, and they're usually willing to have a discussion with non-profit leagues, like those that are designed for youth athletics, in order to make the costs manageable. When planning to bring these sorts of outside groups to the attention of the association, be sure to have decided on a way to ensure there are no extra costs that will be borne upon the association or the players and their families; the need is to provide a service that has to be given to all players and without increasing the financial burden to those families, many of whom will not understand the need for the policy change and the need for these outside groups to come in to work with the teams. On the other hand, most sports organizations are used to having outside groups come in and work with their players, and there are often ways of ensuring that those benefits are passed onto the players without having additional costs be added. When I played baseball we would often have professional coaches from a local training program join the team and there were never and financial penalties associated with having these experts work with the team, they were just there and the association either had a fund in place devoted to providing these kinds of programs to players, or the training program itself offered to work with the team at a reduced cost or for free. There was never any point where my parents or I were required or requested to pay extra to attend or to subsidize those who did attend, as these extra clinics were primarily for the pitching and catching staff.

It's important to note also that these potential partner groups are not meant to supplant the efforts of the association itself; it's all well and good to have these outside groups come in and lecture about the need for greater tolerance, but it won't mean anything if the association doesn't stand behind that message and act on its own without those groups. So yes, while it can be of benefit to invite these groups to participate in your association and provide insights to your board and the players about why transphobia and homophobia are problematic in the locker room or field, those lessons are best learned by showing an internal commitment to continuing those lesson once the outside groups have left for the evening. This means that even after the groups come in and do their presentation with the players or board members or coaches, there will need to be written policy changes that accentuate what's been learned in the presentations or workshops done with the outside queer advocacy groups that are brought in to meet with your association, and there will also be enforcement of those policy changes once they're put into place. The whole process is going to take far more than the one year that the presentations are made and the first board accepts making those changes, it's going to include constant work to ensure that future boards are put in place that are willing to accept the new policy and make sure that those policies are upheld, which could mean having those outside groups come back to discuss issues of queer equality with the coaching staff each and every year. That too is something that can be addressed and decided once the organization feels comfortable with the idea of bringing in a group to talk with some of their members.

Within most organizations, the main problem with creating new policies or changing old policies is the speed in which any kind of change is going to occur. This is not a phenomenon specific to changes in policy that would protect queer youth in their sports organizations; most non-profit groups and other bodies that work with a board of directors are slow to implement policy due to institutional barriers that require the board or its representatives to obtain feedback and the permission of the membership before any changes can be made to the organization. This is usually done to protect the board, which are almost always comprised of volunteers who agree to be part of the organization because of their links to the program. These links the executive have are usually their children who are participants in the organization. This means that these are not normally professionals for whom the board of directors for your sports association is the only thing they do with their day, and in fact it may be something that they do not do for very much of their day or year either. Most people will get onto board like these thinking that they will be part time affairs and fully based on administering to the needs of the players, which is not something they expect will need a large investment of their time. For the most part, this is correct; even people on the executive find that they do not have that much to do once the season is underway and the main logistical and administrative components of the job have been completed. However, this means that these executives are not often interested or willing to create wholesale changes that will affect the organization after they have left their position as board members, often because they lack the expertise needed to execute those changes after they have been approved by the organization's membership.

These executives also do not generally have the inclination to undergo a major policy change in their organizations, as their main goal is to facilitate the everyday operations of the league and ensuring that participants' needs are taken care of with respect to insurance, facility bookings and ensuring the teams associated with the organization are qualified and certified to participate in interclub league play with other organizations in the surrounding area. These needs are the primary concern for the organization executive and very often leave little time for the pursuit of other goals, even ones that may help expand or protect the membership of the organization. Many of these sports organizations also lack the capacity to undergo the kinds of feedback and consultation that would be needed to achieve the cooperation and buy-in of the membership, which would be critical to the success of any policy change that the organization might wish to undertake.

This lack of ability to effectively consult with the organization's membership is based on and a symptom of the way these organizations are run; there's only ever activity during the sports season, and once the season is over the organization does not have any activities they need to undertake. This lack of off-season activity means that there's no need to continue outreach to the members, and in turn usually means that there are limited numbers of people interested in attending annual general meetings and bringing new ideas or policies to the group for ratification or discussion. What is created is a cyclical problem where there's no ability for the executive or board to interact with the members, which in turn means there is no interest in becoming part of the board or presenting new ideas to them for discussion with the rest of the group. In the case of creating policies that would protect queer youth while they participate in athletics as part of their organization, this creates a problem where the concerns of queer youth can never be heard, and if they are heard then there is no way to canvass more opinions and ensure that the views of those queer youth and their families is representative of the organization as a whole and will be accepted by the rest of the members.

The final concern with the policymaking process as it relates to youth athletics organizations is the simple fact that many of the people who serve on these boards of directors both do not understand there is a problem and do not know how to fix the problem. These men and women are well intentioned and are likely to want to help make their organization safe for all potential participants, but for many of them the issue is so far removed from their daily lives that they do not understand how to be a helpful ally. This is difficult for many activists and youth to understand, as this lack of understanding of the issues can be interpreted as opposition to the concept of creating queer-friendly policies. This ambivalence can be addressed by youth themselves by discussing the impact a potential change in policy would have on them on a personal level, and in sharing stories of how the current policy system is not working for the youth already part of the organization.

What these concerns normally reduce to are a lack of communication between the members of the association during the off season and the unwillingness to do anything outside of working on the needs of the teams and players during the season itself. There is very little consultation that goes on and there are no experts within the organization that are able to roll out these kinds of policy changes that would have to be put in place to create safer spaces for queer players. A lot of this is also based on the relatively quick turnaround of most members of the association's executive; most people find that they are only interested in volunteering for a single year, and then they move on or let other people take their turn. This means that there is often very little in terms of institutional memory of the discussions you may have had with other executives about changing the policy, and effectively means that each year the policy is not created is another year that will be reset once the new board comes in. This mounting frustration can mean that even those dedicated to pursuing non-discrimination policies may become too exhausted and frustrated by the lack of movement to complete the policy change, or that the people who initially made the complaint in order to draw attention to the problem will have long left the program, either because they are no longer able to participate safely or because they have aged out of the program itself.

Even in situations where there remain people who stay as part of the organization's executive for multiple years, they often do so because of their expertise in the actual running of the organization, as opposed to their ability to create policies or otherwise push through the kinds of changes that are likely to be asked for by players that have faced discrimination in the league. This often means that instead of leaving the policy creation to the board of directors, it becomes necessary to create a policy or series of potential draft policies that can already be selected and voted upon, and then to volunteer to help create the infrastructure needed to ensure those policies are executed properly. When attempting to create the policy 5.45 in the Burnaby school district, a lot of the work was done by the outside group trying to conceive of the policy. We looked at draft policies that were used by other school districts and used those as templates for policies that we could bring to the board for discussion, instead of adding to their workload by telling them that we wanted a policy and that they would also have to create it without any help from the people who wanted that policy to be created.

Having these draft policies available also makes it easier to obtain support from the rest of the organization. Too often it's easy to support or oppose an abstract idea, either because it seem acceptable in principle or because people are able to conjure up what they believe will be a significant logistical challenge that the organization is not capable of executing along with their duties to the players to ensure that the athletics themselves are able to occur without any outside problems. Having explicit plans for what you intend to do will show people that there's no hidden agenda to go further than the changes needed to create safe spaces, and by having a plan that shows what you would be attempting to do and how it would work out, it also shows that there's been more initiative taken than simply demanding something; it shows that the logistical concerns and other potential problems have been addressed and that they are surmountable without compromising the rest of the organization. This will make it more likely to become supported by more people when first presenting the proposal to the board.

These draft policies will also help during the consultation phase of the policy creation process. Once people have something that is concrete and could be enacted, an actionable set of ideas, there becomes a much more useful conversation than a simple conversation about the viability of doing something at all. People involved with the organization are more likely to be supportive of a policy change once they can see how it would look and what the effects would be, and they can also provide input as to how those processes could be streamlined once they are put into effect. That's a better conversation to be having than the conversation about whether there should be any policy change at all, and is more constructive than consultation sessions devoted to multiple different versions of what different people believe should happen; they'll have the one plan available to them and they can either support it or not support it, which will save time that would otherwise be spent trying to hear what everyone's views are and then synthesize them into a single coherent viewpoint, which often won't happen at all if there are many voices opposed to the creation of any policy. Their views would have to be taken into account and that could mean that the policy you wish to have enacted could be made less effective to take into consideration the views of people who are not interested in helping you.

Before I was born, if you told someone that you were gay you were publicly ridiculed and even considered to be carrying a mental disease that could make you a danger to yourself and the rest of society. After I was born, to be gay was to live a lifetime in the closet and to stay quiet about who you were. Considering joining an athletics organization or participating in sports of any kind as a gay person meant that you had to be incredibly deep in the closet, even if you were considered one of the best at your sport. There were always going to be people that were known to be queer and involved in sports, but most would never admit to it until after their careers were over, or they were considered an outlier that was not meant to be repeated or acknowledged by anyone as worth thinking about. This was the culture of the time in which I was born and the time preceding my life, and it serves as a reminder of just how far we have come in North American society to go from a complete lack of understanding as to how people came to identify as part of the queer continuum and using us as stereotypes and scapegoats to where we have come so far, where people are generally accepting and in most cases are willing to treat queer people with respect and understanding. Even after I started growing up, being openly queer was hard to do and not something that you would ever consider as part of a sane childhood, especially if you had any aspirations of being involved in sports. First, you would have been stereotyped and people would not have believed you would have had any interest in sports to begin with, something that is continuing to lead queer youth away from athletics even for those who do have an interest. Even if you could get beyond this kind of stereotyping and intolerant thinking, there would have been the commentary and abuse that teammates and opponents would hurl your way once you were on the field that you would have to deal with as an openly queer player. It made it difficult growing up to be the only queer player I knew, and it was enough that for most of my own career I hid that part of who I was from the people I played with, even though doing so harmed my game and objectively made me a less talented player on the field and on the ice.

Who would have thought that even a short decade after my youth sports career started to take off that we would have professional and collegiate athletes coming out and telling the whole world that they were queer, and not only that they were queer but that they remained some of the very best athletes in their sports. The increasing numbers of athletes coming out has prompted a whole new field of athletics reporting and new areas to research and develop in our athletic training programs. Queer athletes have many of the same issues and concerns that their heterosexual peers have to deal with in their daily lives, but there are many issues that will arise with queer athletes that will be totally unique and that coaches and other support personnel need to be aware of. This means that entirely new training programs need to be created to address these incoming needs. These athletes who come out while participating are always going to be a tiny minority of the athletics population, and like all minorities this means this puts them in a vulnerable position among their peers. It's what kept me from coming out for most of my sports career as a youth; I was too concerned about how I would potentially be treated by my teammates. But that was because I was alone and didn't even know there were other out queer athletes in existence, and certainly not that some were professional athletes. Knowing that might have let me come out earlier in my life, instead of waiting until nearly the end of my athletics career to do so.

That was then. Now it's becoming less of an issue to be queer, not just in society as a whole but in athletics as well. There's no longer the feeling of being totally isolated or alone, because technology has made it easier than ever to find stories and examples of other queer athletes around the world. These stories and examples from around the world help us remember that we're not alone, and it provides a different kind of support for queer athletes that didn't exist prior to the explosive growth of the internet. It isn't just that queer youth can use the internet to find examples of other queer youth; our municipalities and local areas are beginning to fill up with all manner of programs that are specifically for queer youth. Even in places where queer-only or queer-friendly leagues don't exist, increasing numbers of queer youth are coming out and finding each other through more traditional sports leagues. More and more, queer youth are becoming increasingly interconnected to each other through athletics. This breaking down of barriers in athletics has continually meant that better health outcomes are becoming part of the new queer youth identity.

Leaving the closets and the clubs behind has been one of the most lasting benefits of engaging queer youth in athletics. Before sports, the easiest way to have a social life was to become part of the club scene and to engage in reckless behaviour. This lifestyle continues to exist to this very day, but its become seen as less popular among younger queers, particularly those who become part of the queer community in other ways. This need to find a community to belong to is one of our most primal instincts, and it was important for me to have sports as my main social outlet as it fulfilled me in ways my other social diversions were not able to do so for me.

In the end, sports and athletics are more than just tests of physical skills and personal training. Sports were and remain a key means of interacting with my social peers and building a sense of community for myself within the greater world around me. It has been through sports that I built strong friendships and developed the personality traits needed to grow and thrive in the world, even when the world seems intent on frustrating or harming me in other endeavours. There may be other ways to grow and develop as a person in contemporary society, but there was no better way for me to become a well-rounded human being than by being involved in sports, and this is a gift that I hope all queer youth are able to share with me in the future.

[i] Wellard, I. (2009). Transcending the heteronormative in sport: masculine sporting

identities, sexualities and in/excusive practices. Retrieved March/14, 2014, from

http://www.revue-quasimodo.org/PDFs/SH-IanWellard.pdf

[ii] Wellard, I. (2009). Transcending the heteronormative in sport: masculine sporting

identities, sexualities and in/excusive practices. Retrieved March/14, 2014, from

http://www.revue-quasimodo.org/PDFs/SH-IanWellard.pdf

[iii] The Associated Press. (2014). Retrieved March/12, 2014, from

http://www.cbc.ca/news/world/vladimir-putin-links-gays-to-pedophiles-1.2502885

[iv] The Associated Press. (2014). Retrieved March 1, 2014, from

http://www.cbc.ca/news/world/yoweri-museveni-uganda-s-president-set-to-sign-antigay-bill-1.2548301

[v] Buzinski, J. (2014). Retrieved March/11, 2014, from

http://www.outsports.com/2014/3/12/5499530/nets-to-sign-jason-collins-for-rest-ofseason

[vi] Buzinski, J. (2014). Retrieved March/11, 2014, from

http://www.outsports.com/2014/3/12/5499530/nets-to-sign-jason-collins-for-rest-ofseason

[vii] Saad, L. (2013). Retrieved March/13, 2014, from

http://www.gallup.com/poll/163730/back-law-legalize-gay-marriage-states.aspx

[viii] Seigler, C. (2014). Retrieved March/12, 2014,

fromhttp://www.outsports.com/2014/2/24/5443428/matt-kaplon-gay-drew-universitybaseball

[ix] Seigler, C. (2014). Retrieved March/12, 2014,

fromhttp://www.outsports.com/2014/2/24/5443428/matt-kaplon-gay-drew-universitybaseball

[x] Buzinski, J., & Zeigler, C. (2007). The outsports revolution (1st ed.). New York, New

York: Alyson Books.

[xi] You Can Play Project. (2013). Retrieved March/11, 2014, from

http://youcanplayproject.org/pages/our-cause

[xii] Toronto Blue Jays. (2014). Retrieved March/15, 2014, from

http://toronto.bluejays.mlb.com/tor/baseball_academy/index.jsp

Bibliography

Buzinski, J. (2014). Retrieved March/11, 2014, from

http://www.outsports.com/2014/3/12/5499530/nets-to-sign-jason-collins-for-rest-ofseason

Buzinski, J., & Zeigler, C. (2007). The outsports revolution (1st ed.). New York, New

York: Alyson Books.

Saad, L. (2013). Retrieved March/13, 2014, from

http://www.gallup.com/poll/163730/back-law-legalize-gay-marriage-states.aspx

Seigler, C. (2014). Retrieved March/12, 2014, from

http://www.outsports.com/2014/2/24/5443428/matt-kaplon-gay-drew-universitybaseball

The Associated Press. (2014). Retrieved March/12, 2014,

fromhttp://www.cbc.ca/news/world/vladimir-putin-links-gays-to-pedophiles1.2502885

The Associated Press. (2014). Retrieved March 1, 2014, from

http://www.cbc.ca/news/world/yoweri-museveni-uganda-s-president-set-to-sign-antigay-bill-1.2548301

Toronto Blue Jays. (2014). Retrieved March/15, 2014, from

http://toronto.bluejays.mlb.com/tor/baseball_academy/index.jsp

Wellard, I. (2009). Transcending the heteronormative in sport: masculine sporting identities, sexualities and in/excusive practices. Retrieved March/14, 2014, from

http://www.revue-quasimodo.org/PDFs/SH-IanWellard.pdf

You Can Play Project. (2013). Retrieved March/11, 2014, from

http://youcanplayproject.org/pages/our-cause

www.ingramcontent.com/pod-product-compliance
Lightning Source LLC
Chambersburg PA
CBHW020318290526
45785CB00007B/2837